Improving Childhood Asthma Outcomes
in the
United States

A Blueprint for Policy Action

A Description of Group Process Methods
Used to Generate Committee Recommendations

Will Nicholas ◆ Marielena Lara ◆ Sally C. Morton

Supported by the Robert Wood Johnson Foundation

RAND

The research described in this report was sponsored by the Robert Wood Johnson Foundation.

Library of Congress Cataloging-in-Publication Data

Nicholas, Will, 1967–
  Improving childhood asthma outcomes in the United States : a blueprint for policy
action : a description of group process methods used to generate committee
recommendations / Will Nicholas, Marielena Lara, Sally C. Morton.
    p. cm.
  "MR-1330/1."
  Includes bibliographical references.
  ISBN 0-8330-3146-5
  1. Asthma in children—Government policy—United States. I. Lara, Marielena. II.
Morton, Sally C. III. Title.

RJ436.A8 N534 2002
362.1'9892238'00973—dc21

                                                                      2002024815

A profile of RAND Health, abstracts of its publications, and ordering information can be found on the RAND Health home page at www.rand.org/health.

RAND is a nonprofit institution that helps improve policy and decisionmaking through research and analysis. RAND® is a registered trademark. RAND's publications do not necessarily reflect the opinions or policies of its research sponsors.

Published 2002 by RAND
1700 Main Street, P.O. Box 2138, Santa Monica, CA 90407-2138
1200 South Hayes Street, Arlington, VA 22202-5050
201 North Craig Street, Suite 102, Pittsburgh, PA 15213-1516
RAND URL: http://www.rand.org/
To order RAND documents or to obtain additional information,
contact Distribution Services: Telephone: (310) 451-7002;
Fax: (310) 451-6915; Internet: order@rand.org

Preface

This report describes the group process used to arrive at the policy recommendations proposed in *Improving Childhood Asthma Outcomes in the United States: A Blueprint for Policy Action*, by M. Lara, W. Nicholas, S. Morton, M. Vaiana, B. Genovese, and G. Rachelefsky, Santa Monica, Calif.: RAND, MR-1330-RWJ, 2001. That report summarizes the findings of an effort funded by the Robert Wood Johnson Foundation, to

- Identify a range of policy actions in both the public and private sectors that could improve childhood asthma outcomes nationwide

- Select a subset of policies to create a blueprint for national policy in this area

- Outline alternatives to implement these policies that build on prior efforts.

Over the course of 2000, RAND Health engaged an interdisciplinary committee of nationally recognized leaders in childhood asthma in a structured group process to identify the policy recommendations in the *Blueprint*. Appendix A provides a schematic of the group process, and this report describes the process in detail. The extensive appendices contain the essential "live" documents (lists, voting sheets, Power Point slides, Excel spreadsheets, etc.) that facilitated this process.

This effort is part of the Robert Wood Johnson Foundation's Pediatric Asthma Initiative. The purpose of this initiative is to address current gaps in national childhood asthma care through clinical and nonclinical approaches to improve the management of childhood asthma. It is the first national initiative that simultaneously addresses treatment, policy, and financing issues for children with asthma at the patient, provider, and institutional levels.

The report is based on research conducted under the auspices of RAND Health. RAND Health furthers RAND's mission of helping improve policy and decisionmaking through research and analysis, by working to improve health care systems and advance understanding of how the organizing and financing of care affect costs, quality, and access.

Contents

Introduction

This report describes the group process used to arrive at the policy recommendations proposed in *Improving Childhood Asthma Outcomes in the United States: A Blueprint for Policy Action*.[1] The latter report summarizes the findings of an effort funded by the Robert Wood Johnson Foundation, to

- Identify a range of policy actions in both the public and private sectors that could improve childhood asthma outcomes nationwide

- Select a subset of policies to create a blueprint for national policy in this area

- Outline alternatives to implement these policies that build on prior efforts.

Over the course of 2000, RAND Health engaged an interdisciplinary committee of nationally recognized leaders in childhood asthma in a structured group process to identify the policy recommendations in the *Blueprint*. Appendix A provides a schematic of the group process, and this report describes the process in detail. The extensive appendices contain the essential "live" documents (lists, voting sheets, Power Point slides, Excel spreadsheets, etc.) that facilitated this process.

This effort is part of the Robert Wood Johnson Foundation's Pediatric Asthma Initiative. The purpose of this initiative is to address current gaps in national childhood asthma care through clinical and nonclinical approaches to improve the management of childhood asthma. It is the first national initiative that simultaneously addresses treatment, policy, and financing issues for children with asthma at the patient, provider, and institutional levels.

---

[1]Lara, M., W. Nicholas, S. Morton, M. Vaiana, B. Genovese, and G. Rachelefsky, *Improving Childhood Asthma Outcomes in the United States: A Blueprint for Policy Action*, Santa Monica, Calif.: RAND, MR-1330-RWJ, 2001.

Description of Group Process Methods

Selection of the Expert Committee

We began the committee selection process by seeking two committee chairs. These chairs would be nationally prominent experts with first-hand knowledge of economic and policy issues related to asthma, and current or prior clinical experience with asthma. We solicited nominations from national asthma organizations and professional and other health care and policy organizations. Drs. Steve Redd and Kevin Weiss agreed to chair the expert committee and participated actively with the research team in all stages of the project, including selection of the other members of the expert committee.

We used a similar process to identify an interdisciplinary group of six additional committee members. We sought individuals with expertise in (1) asthma education and community outreach, (2) delivery of asthma health care services in diverse settings, (3) environmental assessment and control, (4) epidemiology and surveillance, (5) health care finance, and (6) government programs and policy. We balanced geographic and gender representation on the committee. The targeted number of committee members was based on an analysis of small groups suggesting that it is difficult to have a meaningful discussion among more than 12 persons.[1] A list of the expert committee members and RAND Health staff can be found in Appendix B. Throughout the group process, the voting group consisted of the eight expert committee members, along with the project's principal investigator and co-principal investigator, for a total of 10 voters.[2]

Construction of a Preliminary List of Policy Levers

The first step in our group process consisted of the construction of a preliminary list of policy levers. We defined a *lever* as an action that could be taken in the public or private policy realm to improve childhood asthma outcomes in the United States.

We based our preliminary list of policy levers on a review of asthma-related publications familiar to the RAND staff and expert committee. The committee members agreed a priori that policy levers should be grouped into five content areas: (1) population-based surveillance, (2) environmental assessment and control, (3) health care organization and delivery, (4) education,

---

[1] Brook, R., "The RAND/UCLA Appropriateness Method," in K. A. McCormick, ed., *Clinical Practice Guidelines Development: Methodology Perspectives,* Rockville, Md.: Department of Health and Human Services, Public Health Services, Agency for Health Care Policy and Research, DHHS/PHS/AHCPR No. 95-0009, 1994, pp. 59–70; Jones, J., and D. Hunter, "Consensus Methods for Medical and Health Services Research," *BMJ* (Clinical Research Ed.), Vol. 311, No. 7001, 1995, pp. 376–380; and Lara, M., and C. Goodman, *National Priorities for the Assessment of Clinical Conditions and Medical Technologies: Report of a Pilot Study,* Washington, D.C.: National Academy Press, Institute of Medicine Publication IOM-89-14, 1990.

[2] Please note that the revised list of 63 policy levers in Appendix F was rated by 11 people. One other expert committee member participated in this rating exercise but subsequently resigned from the committee.

and (5) financing and regulation. Within each content area, policy levers were chosen according to five priority-setting criteria:

- **Feasibility of implementation.** How feasible would the implementation of this lever be? Would the necessary resources be available? Would it be politically viable? Could this policy lever be carried out in the real world?

- **Support by evidence.** To what degree would this lever be supported by research or historical evidence? Have well-controlled trials been conducted in representative populations? If not, would emerging research or expert judgment support effectiveness?

- **Reduction of inequalities.** Would this lever reduce inequalities in asthma outcomes among underserved children? If implemented, would this lever reduce health care delivery barriers and other risk factors that disproportionately affect vulnerable populations?

- **Reduction of net costs.** Would this lever be cost-effective? After including cost for implementation, would this lever reduce overall societal costs for asthma?

- **Improvement of overall outcomes.** Would this lever improve childhood asthma health-related outcomes? Would it reduce symptom burden and improve child and family quality of life? Would it reduce preventable asthma hospitalizations and deaths?

Our preliminary list consisted of 57 policy levers, which we distributed to the entire committee for review. We solicited members' comments via a semi-structured feedback form (see Appendix C). Given feedback received from all committee members, we generated a document listing each of the original 57 levers, followed by member-generated pros and cons and descriptions of suggested revisions made to arrive at a new list of 63 levers (see Appendix D). During this stage, the committee members decided to add "research" to the list of five policy content areas (population-based surveillance, environmental assessment and control, etc.).

Member Rating of Revised List of 63 Policy Levers

We then conducted a rating of the revised list of 63 policy levers by mail. We asked committee members to rate each of the 63 levers across the five priority-setting criteria described above. In addition, the members were asked to assign an overall grade of A, B, C, or D to each lever (in the subsequent analysis, an A was considered a score of 4; B, a score of 3; C, a score of 2; and D, a score of 1). Appendix E contains the rating instructions and ballot.

Analysis of the Ratings

We entered the rating data into Excel for analysis. Appendix F contains the results of the analysis, along with explanatory notes. An algorithm determined a priori, in consultation with committee chairs, was applied to the analysis results to determine the top set of levers. The algorithm identified those levers *in the top 20 of the 63 levers* by average overall grade, *and in the top two-thirds on all five priority-setting criteria* (feasibility, evidence, inequalities, costs, and outcomes). Seventeen levers met these criteria: 2 in the population-based surveillance content area, 2 in environmental assessment and control, 4 in health care organization and delivery, 6 in education, 2 in financing and regulation, and 1 in research. These 17 levers are shaded in the analysis results presented in Appendix F.

Meeting Agenda

Before the meeting, the committee members were sent the results of the rating exercise, along with all qualitative comments collected on the rating ballot. The objective of the meeting, as defined by the project team and committee chairs, was to come up with a "top-10" list of policy recommendations. We started the meeting with a discussion of the policy levers in each content area. For this discussion, we focused on those levers in each area that were among the 17 that met the pre-meeting algorithm criteria (see above). However, we allowed committee members a final opportunity to argue for the inclusion of *any* of the 63 levers. To facilitate this initial discussion, we presented the individual committee members with overheads summarizing the ratings within each content area (see Appendix G).

At the end of this first discussion period, the committee agreed on a list of 21 policy recommendations to be subjected to a final vote. These 21 recommendations consisted of some rewordings of the original levers, as well as some collapsing of two or three related levers into a single policy recommendation (see Appendix H).

Each committee member was asked to vote for 10 of the 21 recommendations to be included in the final report.[3] To reach our goal of 10 recommendations, we began by eliminating those recommendations that received less than three votes. This left us with 14. We then combined a few related levers to come up with a final list of 11. Appendix H contains the ballot of 21 recommendations, along with their relationships to the revised list of 63 policy levers and the final list of 11 policy recommendations. For example, the lever in the first row is a combination of original levers 1, 3, and 4, and is contained in final policy recommendation 10.

During the second day of the meeting, we began the process of working together to create a policy framework in which to couch the 11 recommendations. To capture the full range of details voiced by the committee members during the meeting, we also started to flesh out the working versions of our 11 recommendations. Finally, we began to discuss implementation and funding options for each recommendation.

Post-Meeting Activities

During the months following the meeting, we held several phone conferences to continue working on the policy framework, the wording of the 11 recommendations, and the implementation and funding options. To make the report relevant to current legislation, one of the committee members (Dr. Sara Rosenbaum) reviewed asthma-related legislation in the 106th Congress (see Appendix I). Based on this review, we revised recommendation 7 (foster *asthma-friendly* communities and home environments) to reflect ways in which our original recommendation could be addressed through the Children's Health Act of 2000.

The RAND staff then produced a first draft of the report. After initial approval by the committee, we sent this draft to 28 asthma-related professional and lay organizations recommended by the members of the committee as appropriate external reviewers (see Appendix J for a list of the reviewers and organizations). After a follow-up period, we received comments on the draft from all 28 organizations.

---

[3] One member participated in the meeting discussion by phone and did not vote.

The RAND staff read through all comments and suggestions received. The majority of comments by the 28 external reviewers did not involve substantive changes to the recommendations. The RAND staff reviewed those comments and incorporated almost all of them into various sections of the report.

The RAND staff then highlighted the 15 specific suggestions that involved substantive changes to the recommendations agreed upon by the committee. The committee members agreed unanimously with nine of these suggestions. There was some disagreement on the other six, so the committee members were asked to vote on them by choosing from a list of options for each (see Appendix K). Options receiving at least 75-percent support among the committee were incorporated into the final report. Only one of the six suggestions received less than 75-percent support on all options. We crafted a compromise position in this case, and the committee approved it unanimously.

Appendix A
Schematic Diagram of Committee Process

RAND team constructs draft list of policy levers based on literature and committee input.

↓

Preliminary List of 57 Policy Levers

↓

RAND project team elicits comments from committee members via semi-structured feedback form.

↓

Revised List of 63 Policy Levers

↓

Committee rates revised list via mail using five priority-setting criteria.

RAND staff applies algorithm to the ratings to identify the top levers.

↓

17 Policy Levers Meeting Algorithm Criteria

↓

Committee meets and has a first round of discussion guided by results of rating exercise.

↓

Newly Revised List of 21 Policy Levers

↓

Committee votes on top ten levers from among 21

Final List of 11 Policy Levers

↓

Committee and RAND team meet several times to translate final 11 levers into detailed recommendations with implementation and funding options.

Appendix B
National Expert Committee Members and Rand Health Staff[1]

National Expert Committee Members

Stephen Redd
Committee Co-Chair
Chief, Air Pollution and Respiratory
Health Branch
Centers for Disease Control and Prevention

Noreen Clark
Dean, Marshall H. Becker Professor of
Public Health
University of Michigan

Nicole Lurie
(Formerly) Principal Deputy Assistant
Secretary for Health
Department of Health and Human Services

Thomas Platts-Mills
Director, Asthma and Allergic Diseases
Center
University of Virginia

Kevin Weiss
Committee Co-Chair
Director, Center for Healthcare Studies
Northwestern Medical School

Sara Rosenbaum
Director, Center for Health Services Research and
Policy
The George Washington University School of Public
Health and Health Services

Vernon Smith
Principal
Health Management Associates

Lani Wheeler
Pediatric and School Health Consultant
Anne Arundel County Department of Health
Maryland

RAND Health Staff

Marielena Lara
Principal Investigator

Gary Rachelefsky
Co-Principal Investigator
Allergy Research Foundation

Sally Morton
Head, Statistics Group

Mary E. Vaiana
Communications Director

Will Nicholas
Associate Policy Analyst

Marian Branch
Editor

Barbara Genovese
Project Manager

**Carolyn Rogers and
Alaida Rodríguez**
Administrative Assistants

---

[1]This appendix appears as part of Marielena Lara et al., *Improving Childhood Asthma Outcomes in the United States: A Blueprint for Policy Action*, Santa Monica, Calif.: RAND, MR-1330-RWJ, 2001.

_____

Name of Reviewer

Appendix C

Policy Options to Improve Pediatric Asthma Outcomes in the United States

Committee Member Feedback Form #1

Instructions: Your answers to the following questions will be discussed in our upcoming conference call TO BE SCHEDULED). **Return your short-survey either by email to** Genovese@Rand.org **or by fax (310) 451-6917 by MAY 15, 2000.** To answer the following questions please refer to the attached **"Project Summary and Draft List of Possible Policy Levers."** **If you have any questions or concerns please call or email Marielena Lara at (310) 393-0411, ext. 7657;** Lara@Rand.org.

1. Please choose **any 10** policy levers from the attached list [see Appendix D] that you would like to comment on. You may select levers in your area of expertise if you wish. If you prefer to review the policy levers in another format please provide your comments in question # 6 below.

Policy Lever #	Does this Lever have Face Validity?	Do You Know of Evidence Supporting It?	Other Comments/ Suggested Revisions

Question 1 (continued)

Policy Lever #	Does this Lever have Face Validity?	Do You Know of Evidence Supporting it?	Other Comments/ Suggested Revisions

2. Please list the number of the policy lever(s) you would delete and state your reason(s) for deletion.

Policy Lever # to Delete	Rationale

3. Please state policy levers you would add and your reason(s) for addition.

Policy Lever to Add	Rationale

4. Please evaluate the attached "**Description of Project Phases**" and "**Conceptual Framework for Candidate Policy Areas.**" How would you modify it?

5. Please list 5-10 published articles or other respected sources we should review or consult with to: a) fine-tune our approach to develop and rank policy options, and b) complete an adequate review of the available evidence.

Name of First Author or Other Contact	Publication, Year or Organization	Other Important Information

Question 5 (continued)

Name of First Author or Other Contact	Publication, Year or Organization	Other Important Information

6. Other comments:

Appendix D
Summary of Committee Member Feedback on First List of 57 Policy Levers

POPULATION-BASED SURVEILLANCE

1. Congress and state legislators would enact **legislation to fund the creation and operation of asthma-surveillance units at the state and local level.** These units would: a) collect and summarize asthma-specific data from schools and health care organizations and providers, b) coordinate the handling of this information and help make it readily available to the public and parties important to the delivery of asthma health care services.

    Arguments in Favor:
    Surveillance allows for needs assessment, targeting of resources and evaluation of interventions. Funding for local surveillance initiatives would be very welcome.

    Arguments Against/Suggestions:
    Surveillance efforts alone are unlikely to have an immediate or direct impact on asthma severity or control. Surveillance data should be linked to health improvement efforts. School-based data will be difficult to get and of poor quality. Usual sources of asthma data (i.e., hospitals and providers) should be thoroughly mined before new sources (i.e., schools) are tapped. This lever should specify surveillance of trends in hospitalizations. Also, it may be difficult to get Congress to pass this kind of legislation.

    Revisions:
    This lever has been revised to strengthen the link between the collection of surveillance data and their use in health improvement efforts (see Lever P1). An additional lever has been added (see Lever P2) that proposes the investigation of the availability of school-based asthma data and the feasibility of prevalence data collection in this setting. The collection of asthma data from schools has been dropped from all levers in this category.

2. The Centers for Disease Control and Prevention, acting as lead agency within the U.S. Department of Health and Human Services, and in collaboration with other federal and state agencies, would **set standards for asthma-surveillance information.** These standards would specify: a) the types of information regarding asthma-related "sentinel" events--i.e., deaths, near-death events, hospitalizations, emergency department visits, and prolonged school and work absences-- to be collected from public health agencies, health care organizations, and schools, and b) the vehicle and frequency for reporting of this information--e.g., monthly reports to the asthma-surveillance unit(s) from schools and health care organizations.

    Arguments in Favor:
    Standardization improves the quality of surveillance data. Standardization will improve the quality and comparability of regional surveillance efforts.

Arguments Against/Suggestions:
Since all surveillance efforts need to be standardized, this lever should be incorporated into Lever 1. Also, since the CDC already has standards for the collection of asthma surveillance data, this lever may not be necessary. Standards for asthma data should include an indication of asthma severity level.

Revisions:
This lever has been revised to propose additions to current asthma surveillance data standards at the CDC (see Lever P3). Such additions would include standardized indicators of asthma severity to allow for the tracking of high-risk patients.

3. State health departments, working with local asthma-surveillance units, would **conduct more-detailed surveillance of those subgroups or geographic areas that have worse outcomes--i.e., deaths, near-deaths, hospitalizations.** This surveillance would include a survey of risk factors in those populations that are amenable to interventions, such as improved access to asthma care and education, and indoor environmental control.

Arguments in Favor:
Given that asthma affects a variety of populations, a targeted public health approach is the best way to focus efforts on those at greatest risk of poor outcomes. This should be made a funding priority.

Arguments Against/Suggestions:
Identification of these subgroups and geographic areas requires having good local data, which is probably only available for deaths. The next priority should be to build capability for good local hospitalization data. Risk factors included in subgroup surveillance should be based on evidence from NCICAS/NIH outcomes research.

Revisions:
This lever has been revised to propose that risk factors included in targeted surveillance of high risk subgroups and regions be chosen based on the latest research linking such factors to asthma-related outcomes (see Lever P4).

4. Federal and state agencies would **elicit asthma-specific information as part of ongoing national and state-level evaluations of the health of the population.** For example, asthma-specific questions would be appended to national or state telephone surveys, and similar information would be collected through schools and health care organizations.

Arguments in Favor:
Having periodic national asthma-related survey data is an important way to get more detailed data on asthma care processes and outcomes and associated risk and protective factors.

Arguments Against/Suggestions:
Data of this nature is already being collected through the NHIS, NHANES and Behavioral Risk Factor Surveillance System. As with Lever P1, data collection alone

will not have an immediate impact on asthma control. Data from schools will be difficult to get and of poor quality.

<u>Revisions:</u>
This lever has been **DELETED** due to overlap with current data collection efforts and similarities with Lever 1 (see Lever P1).

5. State health departments, working with local agencies, would **conduct sporadic broader-scale screening for asthma.** The screening would ascertain the prevalence of asthma in the population, including possible under diagnosis of mild cases.

    <u>Arguments in Favor:</u>
    Screening for asthma is a good way to assess the problem of under diagnosis on a population level.

    <u>Arguments Against/Suggestions:</u>
    This lever does not add significantly to other levers proposed. Similar data is being collected through other levers. Under diagnosis is an important question from a research standpoint—this would guide surveillance but not be a part of it. There is no clear evidence that screening changes outcomes.

    <u>Revisions:</u>
    This lever has been **DELETED** due to the lack of evidence regarding the feasibility and effectiveness of screening for asthma. This lever has been replaced with a new lever that proposes feasibility and effectiveness research in the area of asthma screening (see Lever O2).

6. State and local asthma-surveillance units, in collaboration with local health providers and health care delivery systems, would **implement mechanisms to identify children who would benefit from early and appropriate asthma care so that progression of the illness could be prevented.** The target population would be children at risk but not yet diagnosed with asthma or children just diagnosed.

    <u>Arguments in Favor:</u>
    Early diagnosis of diseases will theoretically allow for interventions to reduce the severity of future disease outcomes. There is some indirect evidence available that early intervention in pediatric asthma can have an effect on disease progression.

    <u>Arguments Against/Suggestions:</u>
    The evidence is not in on the effects of early asthma intervention. The CAMP study, funded by NHLBI, is looking at this issue. This lever should only be used once the evidence is in. This lever could be integrated with Lever 1, but the decision about how to define "at risk" children is important and difficult. This lever is important from a research standpoint, but it is more a healthcare delivery issue. Children identified this way would be limited to those in contact with health care providers.

Revisions:
This lever has been **DELETED** due to the current lack evidence of the feasibility and effectiveness of early detection and intervention. Lever O2 and other current research are designed to address this lack of evidence.

7. States would enact **legislation requiring evaluation of all children for asthma. Parents** of children entering day care or elementary school would provide certification that their children have been evaluated by a licensed physician for the possible presence of asthma.

Arguments in Favor:
This lever draws on the experience of increased immunization rates when proof of immunization was required for school entry. Widespread evaluation of school-aged children for asthma could lead to the detection of undiagnosed cases and the treatment of newly diagnosed children. Asthma is common enough in this age group to warrant such a screening effort.

Arguments Against/Suggestions:
This is a very expensive unfunded mandate with questionable benefits. There is no validated screening tool for detecting early cases. A disease-of-the-month approach will lead to evaluation of ALL conditions and no good tool will emerge. There is no clear evidence that "screening" changes outcomes.

Revisions:
To address feasibility constraints, this lever has been revised to incorporate asthma evaluation as part of existing school entry health screening (see Lever P5).

8. Local health departments would **conduct a case-by-case investigation of every asthma death and near-death.** Feedback would be given to all parties involved in the care of the patient. Those parties found to be contributory to the event would be reported to the appropriate authorities so that corrective actions would be taken and future deaths prevented.

Arguments in Favor:
Will generate better data upon which to base research. Surveillance alone will not identify risk factors--would need a comparison population.

Arguments Against/Suggestions:
Reviewers commented on several aspects of this lever that needed improvement: This lever should give instructive feedback to family and providers but not be punitive. This is a lot of work for little benefit. Government should not be involved in the evaluation of bad events and punishment of offenders. Policy objectives of the levers should be positive. This is not a very practical lever and there is little evidence to support it. Most local health departments do not have the expertise to conduct this type of investigation. This lever is too narrowly focused. Wording should replace "death" with acute episode or near death. Wording should convey a lower level of investigative effort.

Revisions:
The punitive aspect of this lever has been removed and separate levers have been created for asthma deaths and near deaths so the relative merit of these alternatives can be evaluated (see Levers P6 and P7).

ENVIRONMENTAL CONTROL

9. The Environmental Protection Agency and state environmental agencies, in collaboration with health care provider groups, would **establish minimum standards for an "environmentally friendly" home for a child with asthma.** The standards would include the absence of: a) carpets and other mite-infested household articles, b) cockroaches, and c) wet or mold-prone areas--particularly in the child's bedroom.

    Arguments in Favor:
    The home environment can have an aggravating effect on asthmatics and may play a role in disease development. There is evidence to support a positive effect of allergen avoidance among asthmatics.

    Arguments Against/Suggestions:
    Home environment policy must be linked to remediation funding (Lever 11) and prevention education (Lever 40). These standards should be disseminated to inform and educate parents. This lever is not practical--The EPA is unlikely to do this.

    Revisions:
    This lever has been combined with Lever 11 and Lever 40 to propose a collaborative agenda for promoting safe home environments for children with asthma (see Lever En1).

10. The Health Department, local health care delivery systems, and public and private payers of care would **fund an environmental assessment of the home of every child with asthma who meets certain criteria.** The criteria would include several hospitalizations or a near-death episode. Inspectors certified by the Health Department would conduct the assessment. The results of this assessment, including presence of smoking persons in the household, would be reported back to the health care provider and made part of the medical chart.

    Arguments in Favor:
    The case for environmental assessment of homes where children with severe asthma live is very good.

    Arguments Against/Suggestions:
    The evidence that it is possible to control exposure in the home environment is limited. There is no clear evidence for the value of this recommendation. It is unlikely that payers would see this as a coverable service.

Revisions:
No revisions have been made to this lever (see Lever En2).

11. States would enact **legislation to fund and authorize home-refurbishment assistance to landlords and families of children with asthma.** State and local health and housing departments would provide the assistance. A family would be required to co-pay for additional work needed because it did not maintain the environmental conditions.

Arguments in Favor:
Controlling exposure to allergens in the home environment is not possible without funding for home-refurbishment.

Arguments Against/Suggestions:
This lever is not feasible. Standards (Lever 9), funding for remediation (Lever 11), and preventive education (Lever 40) should all be linked. It is unrealistic to expect legislators to pass this.

Revisions:
Please refer to revisions to Lever 9 (see new Lever En1).

12. Local health and housing departments would **establish regulations for reporting and fining of landlords who do not make medically necessary environmental improvement(s).** Fines collected from landlords would be used to make the environmental improvements.

Arguments in Favor:
It is important to have a mechanism in place that motivates landlords to make necessary environmental improvements to avoid risk of adverse outcomes among children with asthma living in the building(s) in question.

Arguments Against/Suggestions:
This could not be done politically without adding all "constituent diseases". This is not feasible or enforceable. This lever needs to be more specific. It is unclear if these improvements would be required if there were no children with asthma in the home.

Revisions:
This lever has been revised to make environmental improvements required specifically for homes of children with asthma (see Lever En3).

13. Congress and states would enact **legislation to establish and fund similar environmental assessment and refurbishing programs for schools and day care centers.** The assessment would concentrate in areas within schools where children with asthma are more likely to be affected (i.e., classrooms, indoor exercise rooms) and in schools in geographic areas where asthma outcomes are worse.

<u>Arguments in Favor:</u>
Schools have been found to be the source of many asthma triggers. This often is due to the fact that schools are physically deteriorating.

<u>Arguments Against/Suggestions:</u>
Schools boards are limited by tax-caps and back-to-basics mandates. Legislators are more likely to pass funding for assessment than for refurbishment.

<u>Revisions:</u>
No substantive revisions have been made to this lever (see Lever En4).

14. Congress and states would enact **legislation to fund the creation and operation of a free, Health Department-certified smoking-cessation program.** Health care providers and school personnel would refer all smoking persons who live in a household with a child with asthma or who work in a school.

<u>Arguments in Favor:</u>
This lever could tap Tobacco Control Program experience in attempting to implement similar programs. Smoking cessation programs work for many people. There is a lot of data on harmful effects of second hand smoke exposure on persons with asthma. This is feasible since tobacco tax funds could be used.

<u>Arguments Against/Suggestions:</u>
This lever will not have the intended effect. This is important for health in general but provides limited direct benefit for asthma. Should focus on asthma related education. Why would Congress do this, given the state tobacco settlements?

<u>Revisions:</u>
This lever has been revised to propose state-level initiatives using state tobacco tax funds and funds from state tobacco settlements (see Lever En5).

15. Local child-abuse departments would **undertake an evaluation of every household in which a child has had a near-death asthma event and an adult in the household smokes.**

<u>Arguments in Favor:</u>
None provided.

<u>Arguments Against/Suggestions:</u>
All reviewers commented negatively on this lever: This would do harm to families already under the gun. This is another demand on overloaded and under funded state agencies. Government should not be involved in the evaluation of bad events and punishment of offenders. Most local child abuse investigators do not have this expertise. This lever could be negatively perceived. The purpose of and evidence supporting this lever are unclear.

<u>Revisions:</u>
This lever has been **DELETED** due to overwhelming lack of support.

16. Public and private organizations would **fund prospective research to evaluate the effect of intensive in-utero and early-life home environmental control in preventing asthma in at-risk children.** Environmental control would include smoking cessation and elimination of mite and cockroach-infested areas. Children who are at risk include those who have a family history of asthma, were premature, or wheezed in the first year of life.

Arguments in Favor:
Still need to work on prevention. Scientific agenda remains important.

Arguments Against/Suggestions:
Prospective studies need to be designed to evaluate environmental issues, immune response and lifestyle issues together. Evidence at present is not clear about early avoidance. This is only a small piece of a much larger prevention research agenda that should be proposed. The first half of this lever proposes research and the second half proposes environmental control. Is this a policy lever or a research agenda?

Revisions:
This lever's wording has been clarified to indicate that it refers to research (see O3). A new lever has been added (O1) that proposes the need for a broader prevention research agenda.

17. State and local regulatory agencies would **develop standards regarding higher water temperatures for commercial Laundromats.** All Laundromats would be required to display their compliance with these standards. This would facilitate families' capacity to wash sheets and other materials for effective mite-control.

Arguments in Favor:
This lever has face validity and is a good idea.

Arguments Against/Suggestions:
This should be written as a choice for customers at the Laundromat--the water temperature should not be forced on the public. 130 degree water does kill mites but this is an impractical lever with questionable value.

Revisions:
This lever has been revised to give Laundromat customers a choice of water temperatures (see Lever En6).

18. The American Academy of Pediatrics would work with other national groups to **evaluate the tradeoffs of water temperature laws,** i.e. – decreasing risks of burns versus reduction of exposure to mites among children with asthma and allergies.

Arguments in Favor:
This lever has face validity.

Arguments Against/Suggestions:
This lever really says nothing relating to public policy directly. Why isn't this aimed at public health agencies or the appropriate federal agency? There is not enough data to support a positive effect for this lever. See Arguments Against/Suggestions for Lever 17.

Revisions:
This lever has been revised to clarify the AAP's role in national policy related to water temperature(see Lever En7).

19. Public and private payers of care would extend durable medical equipment coverage to mattress and pillow covers.

Arguments in Favor:
This lever has face validity and supporting evidence in literature is increasing.

Arguments Against/Suggestions:
This lever should be moved to financing and regulation. It is not clear whether this alone will help. The slippery slope argument makes this lever unfeasible—what about other environmental modifications? Sofas? Stuffed chairs? Payers will resist covering non-medical items.

Revisions:
This lever has been modified to specify coverage for only those pieces of equipment for which scientific evidence of associations with asthma outcomes is available (see Lever En8).

IMPROVING HEALTH CARE ORGANIZATION AND DELIVERY

20. States would enact **legislation to fund an annual evaluation of any child with asthma who meets certain criteria**. The criteria would include being hospitalized, attending the ED more than 3 times last year, or missing more than 2 weeks of school due to asthma. An interdisciplinary team would conduct this evaluation. The team would include a medical provider with expertise in asthma, a mental health professional, a social worker, and a school liaison. It would set specific treatment and management goals.

Arguments in Favor:
None provided

Arguments Against/Suggestions:
Some 40% of children are on Medicaid/Chip which would fund such services. For those with private insurance this may be covered as medically necessary. It is bad to further fragment care. Why fund separately what should be covered in primary care? This lever should be moved to the financing category.

Revisions:
This lever has been **DELETED** since children with asthma are already being evaluated by health care providers under public and private health insurance plans and the mandate proposed would fragment services. Specific criteria for evaluation and treatment of children with asthma will be incorporated in Levers 27-30 (see new Levers H6-H9). Recommendations for coverage of an interdisciplinary evaluation have been incorporated into levers 45 and 46 (see new Levers F6 and F7).

21. States would enact **legislation requiring health care providers to conduct a comprehensive evaluation at the time of asthma diagnosis and every 5 years thereafter.** As part of this evaluation, specific treatment and management goals would be set. A licensed physician would have to certify that such an evaluation is unnecessary.

    Arguments in Favor:
    None provided.

    Arguments Against/Suggestions:
    This lever is unclear. To be a licensed physician you have to perform these evaluations?

    Revisions:
    This lever has been **DELETED** for the same reasons as Lever 20.

22. National provider and quality-assurance organizations would **establish quality-of-care standards for health care providers who take care of children with asthma.** The standards would be tailored to different settings (ED, hospitalization, outpatient).

    Arguments in Favor:
    There is evidence of low levels of adherence to guidelines and of variability in practice among providers. Care for other conditions has improved with standards.

    Arguments Against/Suggestions:
    Setting standards alone does not ensure adherence. Implementation of guidelines should be done in collaboration with providers and health care organizations.

    Revisions:
    This lever has been **DELETED** because it is not specific enough. Levers 27-30 have been revised to propose national quality standards in each of four separate areas of asthma care (see new Levers H6-H9).

23. Health care systems would **institute quality-improvement strategies to assess and improve the quality of asthma care in different settings, according to national quality-of-care standards.** Quality-improvement standards would include standardized forms, clinical protocols, profiling providers and providing them with this information. The different settings would be EDs, hospitals, and outpatient clinics.

<u>Arguments in Favor:</u>
There is good evidence that quality improvement efforts can change and improve clinical practices in health care organizations.

<u>Arguments Against/Suggestions:</u>
Audit and feedback mechanisms should be added as a QI strategy since they have been shown to be particularly effective.

<u>Revision:</u>
This lever has been revised to include audit and feedback mechanisms as a recommended QI strategy (see Lever H1).

24. Health care delivery systems would **institute electronic or other tracking mechanisms to identify patients with asthma who are uncontrolled.** Criteria for being uncontrolled would include hospitalization, more than 3 ED visits, or more than 2 weeks of school missed due to asthma in the last year. Systems would automatically notify patients and providers of need for evaluation by the primary care provider.

<u>Arguments in Favor:</u>
Automated patient tracking mechanisms can help identify patients in need of asthma related care and managements who would otherwise have fallen through the cracks.

<u>Arguments Against/Suggestions:</u>
This would be an effective strategy for providing technical assistance to providers but should not be used to tell providers how to manage patient care. This should be a voluntary system. This definition of uncontrolled asthma includes too few children. Definition should include children with two or more episodes per week or more than one nighttime symptom per week.

<u>Revisions:</u>
This lever has been revised to clarify that this would be a voluntary system designed to track initially only the most severely uncontrolled cases. Individual organizations could voluntarily elect to broaden their definition of an uncontrolled case (see Lever H2).

25. Health care delivery systems would **institute electronic or other tracking mechanisms to identify patients with asthma needing an evaluation.** The target patients would be those who have not been evaluated for asthma in the past 2 years. The health care delivery system would conduct a family follow-up patient survey to evaluate asthma control and lack of follow-up.

<u>Arguments in Favor:</u>
See Lever 24.

This would be an effective strategy for providing technical assistance to providers but should not be used to tell providers how to manage patient care. This should be a voluntary system. Providers would comply to the extent they saw medical value.

Revisions:
This lever has been revised to propose a voluntary tracking system (see Lever H3).

26. Federal and state governments would **fund the creation of "asthma-provider centers" within local health care delivery system(s).** Health care providers would establish these centers, whose staff would include primary and specialist providers, asthma educators, and case managers. State or local Health Departments would certify the centers. The asthma center staff would: a) be the hub for asthma education for all providers within that geographic area, b) coordinate screening at schools, workplaces, and primary care facilities to obtain asthma population-based surveillance data for that local health care delivery system, c) serve as a referral center to knowledgeable asthma providers, and d) provide care for difficult-to-control children or those children who lack an asthma-trained health care provider.

Arguments in Favor:
The coordination of these various functions in "centers" would centralize valuable asthma community resources.

Arguments Against/Suggestions:
These provider centers would only be beneficial to the extent that patients have access to them. This is only possible if such centers have the capacity to deal with asthma. There is no evidence of the value of such centers.

Revisions:
This lever has been revised to clarify the local asthma center's role in direct health care delivery and how it would work with/supplement asthma surveillance units (see Lever H5).

27. Health care providers would **undertake specific services with each asthma hospitalization.** The services would include the following: a) an asthma physician and case-manager/social worker who would jointly evaluate reasons for admission, b) an asthma educator who would provide the family with information on how the admission could have been prevented and on the regimen of discharge medications and equipment, c) a discharge coordinator who would provide a simple written plan, in the family's language, regarding actions to be taken after discharge, including a follow-up appointment within 1 week of discharge, and d) and the asthma case-manager who would follow up by phone within 3 weeks of discharge to evaluate the child's status and any problems in accessing health care.

Arguments in Favor:
A number of studies have shown the effectiveness of a case-management and patient education/self-management approach to chronic disease care. This approach is also cost-effective.

Arguments Against/Suggestions:
This is not feasible. It is unclear how you would implement this---through licensure mandates? Through mandates in government payer contracts? How to practice medicine has historically worked as education, not as mandates. This lever requires practice protocols and monitoring.

Revisions:
This lever has been revised to propose national quality standards for care related to asthma hospitalizations (see Lever H6).

28. Health care systems would **provide case-management/social worker services to ensure that any child who has had more than 3 asthma hospitalizations in the past 2 years or a near-death episode, and its family, receives primary care by a certified asthma provider.** Care would include an examination by the certified asthma provider at least every 3 months and all necessary medications and equipment ordered by that provider.

Arguments in Favor:
The case management model has been shown to be effective.

Arguments Against/Suggestions:
This should include needed mental health services. Case-management is expensive. This would need to be an item for NCQA, HEDIS or JCAHCO. How to practice medicine has historically worked as education, not as mandates.

Revisions:
This lever has been revised to propose national quality standards for care of children with multiple asthma-related hospitalizations (see Lever H7).

29. Health care providers, in collaboration with local asthma-surveillance units, would **conduct a more in-depth evaluation and treatment plan for each child who survived a near-death episode (ICU admission or history of respiratory arrest).** This process would include an environmental and social evaluation of the household, and 3 monthly home visits by a health care provider to facilitate education, obtaining of medications and equipment, compliance with medication regimen, and household environmental refurbishment.

Arguments in Favor:
This lever has face validity.

Arguments Against/Suggestions:
It is unclear how you would implement this---through licensure mandates? Through mandates in government payer contracts? How to practice medicine has historically worked as education, not as mandates.

Revisions:
This lever has been revised to propose national quality standards for children who have survived an asthma-related near-death episode (see Lever H8).

30. Health care providers would **provide education and case management for all children discharged from the ED for asthma.** Education and case management would include: a) providing in-ED videotape and take-home written instructions regarding regular monitoring of symptoms, appropriate use of equipment and preventive medications, and prompt treatment and follow-up of exacerbations, b) supplying necessary medications and equipment if the family does not have them, c) making a follow-up appointment with an certified asthma provider, and d) notifying the primary provider that the child was seen in the ED for asthma.

Arguments in Favor:
Case management is a cost-effective approach with clear evidence of benefits. Studies of case management in high risk groups suggest positive outcomes.

Arguments Against/Suggestions:
Effect of case-management on asthma ED discharges is not proven. It is unclear how you would implement this---through licensure mandates? Through mandates in government payer contracts? How to practice medicine has historically worked as education, not as mandates.

Revisions:
This lever has been revised to propose national quality standards for all children discharged from the ED for asthma. (see Lever H9).

31. Health care systems would **undertake chart abstraction for children who have been in the ED or missed more than 2 regular appointments for asthma.** The chart abstraction would evaluate the child's risk level. Depending on the risk level, the health care system would institute one of the follow-up algorithms stated above.

Arguments in Favor:
None provided.

Arguments Against/Suggestions:
This lever duplicates lever 24 (electronic tracking systems to identify uncontrolled asthma cases). It is unclear how you would implement this (see Arguments Against/Suggestions for Lever 27)

Revisions:
Due to the similarities between this lever and Levers 24 and 25 (see new Levers H2 and H3), Lever 31 has been **DELETED.**

32. Health care providers would undertake **identification and annual follow-ups of children at risk for asthma.** Identification activities would be part of well child care during the first five years of life. Criteria for being at risk would be family history, prematurity, wheezing in the first year of life, or other suggestive symptoms.

Arguments in Favor:
This lever has face validity.

Arguments Against/Suggestions:
This may already be part of current practice/standard of care. This lever is not feasible because the definition of "at risk" is not clear. This lever could be combined with Lever 6. It is unclear how you would implement this---through licensure mandates? Through mandates in government payer contracts? How to practice medicine has historically worked as education, not as mandates.

Revisions:
This lever has been **DELETED** due to the lack evidence of the feasibility and effectiveness of early detection and intervention. Lever O2 proposes research in this area.

33. Health care systems would **institute pharmacy-based tracking systems to identify patients with asthma who are uncontrolled.** Uncontrolled patients are those who have received more than 2 bronchodilator inhalers in the past month or who have failed to refill an anti-inflammatory medication in the time expected. Automatic referrals for an outpatient evaluation would be sent to the primary asthma provider and the patient's family.

Arguments in Favor:
HEDIS has used pharmacy-based data for quality monitoring. Many systems have this technology in place already.

Arguments Against/Suggestions:
The lever would require the development of appropriate software for tracking patients. The feasibility and financial implications of this should be considered.

Revisions:
No revisions have been made to this lever (see Lever H4).

34. Local asthma centers, schools, and voluntary community groups would **collaborate to institute a combined asthma health care and school-based program for all schools in their geographic area.** This program would facilitate asthma education of school personnel, asthma training of school nurses, referral of children with asthma (particularly those with uncontrolled symptoms) to a local provider, availability of asthma medications and equipment in the schools, and assistance in case of emergencies.

Arguments in Favor:
Research supports the effectiveness of this approach.

Arguments Against/Suggestions:
The approach should be targeted at schools with high rates of asthma. These rates would be determined through school surveillance.

Revisions:
This lever has been revised to propose the targeting of schools in high prevalence areas (see Lever H10).

EDUCATION

35. National asthma, provider, and quality assurance organizations would **set simple, minimal standards for the content of asthma education.** Asthma education would be for patients/families, providers, and school personnel.

     Arguments in Favor:
     This lever has face validity.

     Arguments Against/Suggestions:
     None provided.

     Revisions:
     No revisions have been made to this lever (see Lever Ed1).

36. The U.S. Department of Health and Human Services, in collaboration with other federal and state agencies and national asthma organizations, would **promote early diagnosis, referral, and treatment of patients with asthma through an educational campaign in the national media.** This campaign would also target high-risk populations, such as ethnic minorities and poor individuals with uncontrolled asthma.

     Arguments in Favor:
     A national education campaign is an effective strategy for raising awareness and promoting appropriate treatment. Raising awareness through educational campaigns has a good track record in areas like smoking, seatbelts, drunk driving and safe sex.

     Arguments Against/Suggestions:
     None provided.

     Revisions:
     No revisions have been made to this lever (see Lever Ed2).

37. National sports and athletic organization(s) would undertake an **educational media campaign directed at physical-education teachers, coaches, and other sports personnel.** The campaign would train these personnel to recognize asthma symptoms and the need for medication before exercise, and to administer basic emergency treatment.

     Arguments in Favor:
     Education is an effective way of raising awareness. This campaign should use famous sports figures as spokespersons.

     Arguments Against/Suggestions:
     None provided.

     Revisions:
     This lever has been revised to incorporate the use of professional athletes as spokespersons (see Lever Ed3).

38. National, state, and local school organizations would **implement a broad-based asthma education program for teachers and children.** This program would be part of the science curriculum in elementary school and high school. It would be a series of class lessons aimed at familiarizing students with the symptoms of asthma and with how to be helpful to a person with asthma during an attack. The program would provide awareness of how common the condition is and how children with asthma can lead normal lives.

Arguments in Favor:
Asthma is a big health issue in which schools play a major role.

Arguments Against/Suggestions:
This type of education should not be limited to the science curriculum. It should be a broad-based health education program for teachers and children. The education should be user friendly and available to students of all ages.

Revisions:
No revisions have been made to this lever (see Lever Ed4).

39. Volunteer organizations with special interest and expertise in asthma (e.g., ALA, AAFA) would **promote the implementation of Health Department-certified asthma education and smoking-cessation programs.** These organizations would work with government agencies, health care organizations, and schools in these implementation efforts.

Arguments in Favor:
Smoking cessation is a key issue in inner city asthma. Smoking cessation education works.

Arguments Against/Suggestions:
The question remains whether it should be a local state or federal effort or whether national asthma organizations should take the lead.

Revisions:
This lever has been revised to clarify the lead agencies in this effort (see Lever Ed5).

40. The Department of Housing, in collaboration with landlord and construction associations, would **institute a national education campaign on controlling indoor environmental exposures in children with high-risk asthma.** The campaign would be directed at educating landlords and building industry officials on the importance of exposure-control activities such as removing carpets and exterminating cockroaches.

Arguments in Favor:
This lever has face validity.

Arguments Against/Suggestions:
This lever should be combined with levers 9 and 11. Standards (Lever 9), funding for remediation (Lever 11), and preventive education (Lever 40) should all be linked.

Revisions:
This lever has been combined with Levers 9 and 11 to propose a collaborative agenda for promoting safe home environments for children with asthma (see Lever En1).

41. Health care providers would ensure completion of a standardized basic-education course on asthma by any child newly diagnosed with asthma and his/her family. The course would include information on symptoms, how to use medications and equipment, what to do in case of an attack, and avoidance of asthma triggers. Materials for the program would be simple, interactive, in the family's language, and at the appropriate reading-level.

Arguments in Favor:
There is much evidence of the effectiveness of comprehensive asthma education.

Arguments Against/Suggestions:
It is hard for the provider to ensure that the child/family completes the education course.

Revisions:
This lever has been revised to clarify the health care organization role in providing and tracking the completion of the education (see Lever Ed6).

42. Health care providers would **ensure completion of an asthma education course by all families of high-risk children.** High-risk children have been hospitalized or in the emergency department in the last year, or have had an asthma-related life-threatening episode.

Arguments in Favor:
There is much evidence of the effectiveness of comprehensive asthma education (NCICAS/NIH). It is important to target families with high-risk children.

Arguments Against/Suggestions:
See Arguments Against/Suggestions for Lever 41.

Revisions:
This lever has been revised to clarify the health care organization role in providing and tracking the completion of the education (see Lever Ed7).

43. Local asthma health care centers, in collaboration with local health care systems, would **hold CME-like courses for all primary providers who see pediatric patients with asthma.** These providers would include family physicians, pediatricians, nurse practitioners, respiratory therapists, and pharmacists. Based on the NHLBI National Guidelines, these programs would be simplified, adapted according to the same principles as patient educational programs, and certified by the Health Department.

Arguments in Favor:
None provided.

<u>Arguments Against/Suggestions:</u>
This lever should include follow-up to verify the benefits of the CME courses.
Evidence shows very limited effect of CME on physician practice.

<u>Revisions:</u>
No revisions have been made to this lever (see Lever Ed8).

FINANCE AND REGULATION

44. Private-sector and public-sector insurance programs would **provide affordable and continuous health insurance for all children.** Universal coverage for all children would benefit children with asthma and those who are at risk or undiagnosed. The government would provide insurance, through MediCaid, CHIP, or other means, to those children who are not eligible for other insurance programs.

    <u>Arguments in Favor:</u>
    Universal coverage is the ideal goal and a long term objective. It is better to cover children with asthma through universal rather than categorical programs. Having asthma should not provide special benefits as this creates an incentive to "acquire" a disease diagnosis that may not be applicable.

    <u>Arguments Against/Suggestions:</u>
    This policy lever is ideal but not currently feasible, so incremental approaches to more universal coverage of children, as well as categorical coverage of children with asthma are necessary.

    <u>Revisions:</u>
    A new lever was added proposing expansions of Medicaid/Chip eligibility (see Lever F2). A new lever was added proposing subsidies for working families that have access to employer benefits but can't afford them (see Lever F3). A new lever was added proposing presumptive Medicaid eligibility for children with asthma (see Lever F4). The importance of continuous/uninterrupted coverage is described in Lever 47 (see Lever F5). Original levers 45 and 46 were revised to be considered as supplemental benefits packages for children with asthma (see Levers F6 and F7).

45. All private and public insurance programs would **provide all children with asthma with full coverage with no co-payments for a basic asthma benefits package.** This basic coverage would include age-appropriate emergency and preventive medications, equipment necessary to deliver these medications, 3 "asthma check-up" visits with a regular provider, and an initial evaluation by an interdisciplinary team as outlined above and every 5 years thereafter, unless certified as unnecessary by a licensed physician.

    <u>Arguments in Favor:</u>
    Cost-sharing always has the potential for deterring patient use of preventive services.

Arguments Against/Suggestions:
Insurance companies are unlikely to support 1st dollar coverage with no cost-sharing for preventive services since it doesn't make actuarial sense. Trying to distinguish "asthma" in this way cannot work. This will create confusion for patients, payers and providers and advocates for other diseases will want the same special treatment.

Revisions:
"No" copayment has been changed to "nominal" copayment for preventive services (see Lever F6).

46. All private and public insurance programs would **provide all children with severe asthma with full coverage with no co-payments for an extended asthma benefits package.** Extended-benefit coverage would include an environmental assessment after each hospitalization, an annual evaluation by an interdisciplinary team to set treatment and management goals, and case-management services to coordinate care from multiple programs and sources, to ensure that these goals are met.

Arguments in Favor:
Evidence shows that children with chronic illnesses don't use services "inappropriately" so this argues against cost-sharing for these services.

Arguments Against/Suggestions:
First dollar coverage with no cost-sharing does not make actuarial sense to insurers, thus making this lever unfeasible. Trying to distinguish "asthma" in this way cannot work. Employers and unions that negotiate plans for their employees may not approve of this due to cost considerations.

Revisions:
"No" copayment has been changed to "limited" copayment for extended services (see Lever F7).

47. All private and public insurance programs would **provide uninterrupted health insurance coverage to all children**. For example, every state MediCaid or CHIP program would adopt a 12-month continuous enrollment option so that children with asthma do not experience interrupted insurance coverage. Similar mechanisms would be put in place for private insurance to assure continued insurance coverage when a child changes insurance plans or providers.

Arguments in Favor:
Interruptions in coverage can leave kids with asthma without access to care when they need it the most.

Arguments Against/Suggestions:
None provided.

Revisions:
No revisions have been made to this lever, but it has been listed as one of the specific coverage expansion options (see Lever F5).

48. Insurance programs would **institute co-payment mechanisms that reward families who adhere to preventive care.** For example, families would be charged a co-pay set according to family income, for excessive use of emergency medications or services (e.g., more than 2 bronchodilator inhalers per month, more than 2 ED visits per year). However, if a certified provider submits documentation that the child has severe asthma in spite of adherence to preventive-medication regimens or that the child has attended all his/her regular-provider visits, the family will not be required to pay this co-pay.

Arguments in Favor:
It is important to encourage seeking of preventive services.

Arguments Against/Suggestions:
This lever would penalize patients with excessive use of emergency services when the use of these services is often beyond their control. Also, it would be difficult to verify patient adherence to preventive care.

Revisions:
Lever was reworded to contain a positive incentive for use of preventive services rather than a negative incentive for emergency services (see Lever F8).

49. Private and public payers of care would **create incentive program(s) for providers who comply with preventive and quality-of-care standards.** For example, health providers who comply with these standards would receive financial bonuses (e.g. cash and/or extra vacation days) proportional to the estimated savings associated with decreased hospitalization and ED use rates by their populations.

Arguments in Favor:
There is evidence that provider incentives lead to changes in clinical practice.

Arguments Against/Suggestions:
These kinds of incentives reward providers who take good notes rather that those who provide good care. Evidence linking specific preventive services with reductions in hospitalization and ED utilization may be weak.

Revisions:
Lever was reworded to propose rewarding providers who do a lot of prevention without specifically tying the rewards to the cost offset from reductions in hospitalizations, etc. (see Lever F9).

50. The appropriate national and state agencies would **require that accreditation of hospitals, managed care organizations, and other providers would include evaluation of a minimum, basic set of asthma care related standards.** For example, to receive NCQA accreditation health care systems would furnish documentation of their compliance with HEDIS asthma standards based on review of a random set of medical records.

<u>Arguments in Favor:</u>
Linking accreditation with asthma care standards provides an incentive to health care organizations that wish to maintain relations with major payers.

<u>Arguments Against/Suggestions:</u>
This lever rewards organizations that keep good records rather than those that provide good care.

<u>Revisions:</u>
This lever was revised to base accreditation on observations of the care process or chart reviews (see Lever F10).

51. The appropriate national and state agencies would **provide accreditation for "Asthma Centers of Excellence" within local health care delivery systems according to more specialized standards.** For example, JCHHO would provide special asthma certification status to hospitals with a high volume of asthma-related hospitalizations and emergency department use. To obtain "asthma certification" hospitals would demonstrate adherence to special standards such as minimum number of providers with expertise in asthma (physicians, nurse practitioners, respiratory therapists, asthma educators, and case managers) and quality assurance protocols for asthma care.

<u>Arguments in Favor:</u>
This lever would promote quality asthma care and specialized education and training at key referral centers in the community.

<u>Arguments Against/Suggestions:</u>
Lots of hospitals see a high volume of asthma cases. How do you decide which hospitals are "centers of excellence"? Rewarding hospitals with a high volume of asthma cases provides an incentive to the hospital to keep its asthma admissions high. Not practical or feasible.

<u>Revisions:</u>
Lever was revised to tie accreditation as an "Asthma Center of Excellence" not to the volume of asthma patients, but to the demonstrated capacity of the institution to adhere to the standards set for classification as a "Center of Excellence" (see Lever F11).

52. Private and public payers of care would **require accreditation to provide basic or more specialized asthma services as part of their condition for payment for these services.** For example, all managed care organizations receiving payment for asthma hospitalization and ED care would be required to meet certain minimum educational standards prior to the patient's discharge.

<u>Arguments in Favor:</u>
Conditioning payment on documentation of care processes may encourage the provision of quality care.

Arguments Against/Suggestions:
Wording and mechanism are not clear. Does this mean setting conditions for MCO participation in contracts? This is not practical or feasible. Distinguishing "asthma" in this way cannot work. Advocates for other diseases will want the same special treatment.

Revisions:
No substantive revisions were made to this lever (see Lever F12), but a lever was added that ties payment of plans/providers to the evaluation of claims data as a quality assessment technique (see Lever F18).

53. Health departments would institute a **grading scheme for health care systems and their "asthma-provider centers."** The grading scheme would be based on national or state-level standards for asthma care and would promote compliance with those standards. The grading information would be provided to the public.

Arguments in Favor:
None.

Arguments Against/Suggestions:
None.

Revisions:
No revisions were made to this Lever (see Lever F13).

54. Congress and state legislators would enact **legislation to penalize payers of care who selectively disenroll children who have high utilization of services.** Some children with asthma are hospitalized and use the ED multiple times because of the baseline severity of their illness. Because "high users" can lead to high costs, a health plan may elect to disenroll these children instead of providing primary preventive services that may not lead to less utilization of expensive services. Payers would be held accountable for financial and other costs to the child with asthma and his/her family as a result of the disenrollment.

Arguments in Favor:
This lever has face validity. This kind of broad-based approach (not disease specific) offers the best chance for success.

Arguments Against/Suggestions:
There are occasions when a provider might disenroll a patient with severe uncontrolled asthma from the Medicaid program in order to get enhanced benefits for that patient under SSI. In this case, the payer should not be penalized.

Revisions:
This lever has been revised to allow for the disenrollment from Medicaid of higher service users who qualify for SSI (see Lever F14).

55. States would **develop mechanisms for certification of asthma educators following nationally accepted standards**. For example, certification would be granted through examination or documentation of prior specialist training, or extended working experience with this population. Any health provider or allied health professional (e.g., health educators, social workers, case managers, respiratory therapists) may be eligible for this certification. A state board designated by the state health department would oversee the certification process and its implementation including possible linkage of asthma education certification to reimbursement level of services.

   Arguments in Favor:
   None provided.

   Arguments Against/Suggestions:
   None provided.

   Revisions:
   No revisions were made to this Lever (see Lever F15).

56. The American Boards of Pediatrics, Family Medicine, and other primary child health care providers would **institute an asthma-specific core module in their national certification process**. These modules would include asthma diagnosis, evaluation of symptom control, indication for anti-inflammatory therapy, and key elements regarding patient education (e.g., medication and equipment use and avoidance of asthma triggers.) All diplomates would participate in this core asthma module. Diplomates who by examination score above a certain threshold would receive an asthma certificate that would qualify them as a certified asthma educator (see Lever 55) and experienced provider (see Lever 57).

   Arguments in Favor:
   This lever has face validity. This would improve asthma education of providers.

   Arguments Against/Suggestions:
   None.

   Revisions:
   No substantive revisions have been made to this lever (see Lever F16).

57. Accreditation bodies would **require that all managed care organizations or integrated health care systems providing care for children with asthma have providers "experienced" in pediatric asthma in their networks**. For instance, documentation of at least one annual visit with an "experienced provider" or in consultation with an "experienced provider" would be required for all children with asthma.

   Arguments in Favor:
   This lever has face validity. This would improve asthma care in managed care organizations. This lever has an analogue in HIV care.

41

Arguments Against/Suggestions:
None.

Revisions:
No revisions have been made to this lever (see Lever F17).

Appendix E
Rating Instructions and Ballot

INSTRUCTIONS: For each lever (N=63) complete the ratings in the following seven (7) categories.

Feasibility of Implementation (How feasible would the implementation of this lever be? Are the necessary resources currently or easily available? Is it politically viable? Can this policy lever be carried out in the "real" world?)

1 = very unfeasible   2 = unfeasible   3 = feasible   4 = very feasible

Supported by Evidence (To what degree is this lever supported by research or historical evidence? Have well-controlled trials been conducted in representative populations? If not, does emerging research or expert judgment support effectiveness?)

1 = not supported at all   2 = not supported   3 = supported   4 = strongly supported

Reduce Inequalities (How likely is this lever to reduce inequalities in asthma outcomes among underserved children? If implemented, would this lever reduce health care delivery barriers and other risk factors that disproportionately affect vulnerable populations?)

1 = very unlikely   2 = unlikely   3 = likely   4 = very likely

Reduce Net Costs (How likely is this lever to be cost-effective? After including cost for implementation, would this lever reduce OVERALL societal costs for asthma?)

1 = very unlikely   2 = unlikely   3 = likely   4 = very likely

Improve Overall Outcomes (How likely is this lever to improve OVERALL pediatric asthma outcomes? Would it reduce symptom burden and improve child and family quality of life? Would it reduce preventable asthma hospitalizations and deaths? Please rate as likelihood of global improvement in health outcomes)

1 = very unlikely   2 = unlikely   3 = likely   4 = very likely

Overall Grade (How would you grade this lever? When you weigh the importance of all the previous criteria, what summary rating would you give this lever?)

A = excellent   B = good   D = deficient   F = failed

Confidence in Rating (How confident are you with your rating of this lever? To what degree is your rating based on direct knowledge and/or "real" world experience?)

1 = not at all confident   2 = not confident   3 = confident   4 = very confident

Instructions: Please rate each of the following policy levers on a scale of 1 to 4 according to the criteria listed and defined on the attached Policy Lever Rating Sheet. Please base your ratings on your best expert knowledge and experience and avoid missing data. PLEASE RETURN IN PRE-ADDRESSED FED-EX ENVELOPE BY JUNE 2ND.

Lever	Criteria	Rating	Comments
Example: *The federal/state government would provide insurance for all uninsured children with asthma*	Feasibility of Implementation Supported by Evidence Reduce Inequalities Reduce Net Costs Improve Overall Outcomes Overall Grade Confidence in Rating	3 3 4 4 4 A 3	
Population-Based Surveillance			
P1. Congress and states would enact legislation to fund the creation and operation of asthma-surveillance units at the state and local level. These units would: a) collect and summarize asthma-specific data from health care organizations (e.g. asthma hospitalizations) and ongoing population-based surveys (e.g. NHIS) and b) coordinate data transfer to public and private parties for use in research and service delivery programs aimed at improving asthma care and outcomes. Cross Reference(s): F18	Feasibility of Implementation Supported by Evidence Reduce Inequalities Reduce Net Costs Improve Overall Outcomes Overall Grade Confidence in Rating		
P2. In collaboration with state and local governments, the CDC would evaluate the availability and quality of asthma data from schools. This would include investigation of efforts to obtain asthma prevalence and morbidity estimates (e.g. school days lost) through school-based data collection.	Feasibility of Implementation Supported by Evidence Reduce Inequalities Reduce Net Costs Improve Overall Outcomes Overall Grade Confidence in Rating		
P3. The Centers for Disease Control and Prevention, acting as lead agency within the U.S. Department of Health and Human Services, and in collaboration with other federal and state agencies, would refine their standards for asthma-surveillance data. These standards would include: a) asthma-related "sentinel events" (e.g. hospitalizations, near death events) to be collected from public health agencies and health care organizations and b) other asthma severity indicators to identify high-risk populations.	Feasibility of Implementation Supported by Evidence Reduce Inequalities Reduce Net Costs Improve Overall Outcomes Overall Grade Confidence in Rating		

For your information, cross references have been provided when one or more levers may be related. PLEASE MAKE SURE YOU RATE EACH LEVER INDIVIDUALLY.

Population-Based Surveillance (continued)

Lever		Criteria	Rating	Comments
P4.	State health departments, working with local asthma-surveillance units, would conduct more detailed surveillance of those subgroups or geographic areas that have worse outcomes. Surveillance would include a survey of risk factors that are both amenable to interventions and that have been shown in recent research to be associated with asthma-related outcomes.	Feasibility of Implementation Supported by Evidence Reduce Inequalities Reduce Net Costs Improve Overall Outcomes Overall Grade Confidence in Rating		
P5.	States would enact legislation requiring evaluation of all children for asthma as a prerequisite for school or day care enrollment. As part of the required school entry history and physical exam, parents would provide certification that their children have been evaluated by a licensed physician for the possible presence of asthma.	Feasibility of Implementation Supported by Evidence Reduce Inequalities Reduce Net Costs Improve Overall Outcomes Overall Grade Confidence in Rating		
P6.	Local health departments would conduct a case-by-case investigation of every asthma **death.** Feedback would be given to the patient's family and all health care parties involved. Information gathered in the investigation would be used to help prevent future deaths. Cross Reference(s): P7	Feasibility of Implementation Supported by Evidence Reduce Inequalities Reduce Net Costs Improve Overall Outcomes Overall Grade Confidence in Rating		
P7.	Local health departments would conduct a case-by-case investigation of every asthma **near death.** Feedback would be given to the patient's family and all health care parties involved. Information gathered in the investigation would be used to help prevent future emergencies for the patients in question. Cross Reference(s): P6	Feasibility of Implementation Supported by Evidence Reduce Inequalities Reduce Net Costs Improve Overall Outcomes Overall Grade Confidence in Rating		

46

Lever	Criteria	Rating	Comments
Environmental Assessment and Control			
En1. The Environmental Protection Agency and the Department of Housing and Urban Development would work with local asthma providers and advocacy groups to: a) establish minimum standards for "environmentally friendly" homes, b) provide funding for environmental remediation assistance to landlords and families, and c) educate landlords and building industry officials on the control of indoor environmental exposure for children with asthma.	Feasibility of Implementation		
	Supported by Evidence		
	Reduce Inequalities		
	Reduce Net Costs		
	Improve Overall Outcomes		
	Overall Grade		
	Confidence Rating		

Environmental Assessment and Control

		Feasibility of Implementation	Supported by Evidence	Reduce Inequalities	Reduce Net Costs	Improve Overall Outcomes	Overall Grade	Confidence in Rating
En6.	State and local regulatory agencies would develop standards regarding higher water temperatures for commercial Laundromats. All Laundromats would be required to offer customers the choice of a higher water temperature. This would facilitate families' capacity to wash sheets and other materials for effective mite-control.							
En7.	The American Academy of Pediatrics, working with other national groups, would form a taskforce to evaluate the tradeoffs of current national law limiting water temperature, i.e. – decreasing risks of burns versus reduction of exposure to mites among children with asthma and allergies.							
En8.	Public and private payers of care would extend durable medical equipment coverage to items proven to reduce the exacerbations of asthma. Such items would include mattresses, pillow covers and other items that play an important role in preventing exposure to known allergens.							
	Cross Reference(s): other financing and regulation levers)							
En9.	The Department of Housing and Urban Development would designate low income public housing as "smoke-free" to reduce childhood exposure to second hand smoke. Smoking would only be allowed in designated outdoor areas.							

Improving Health Care Organization and Delivery

	Description	Ratings
H1.	Health care systems would institute quality-improvement strategies to assess and improve the quality of asthma care in different settings, according to national quality-of-care standards. Quality improvement strategies would include standardized forms, clinical protocols, and audit and feedback mechanisms. The different settings would be EDs, hospitals, and outpatient clinics.	Feasibility of Implementation Supported by Evidence Reduce Inequalities Reduce Net Costs Improve Overall Outcomes Overall Grade Confidence in Rating
H2.	Health care delivery systems would institute electronic or other tracking mechanisms to identify patients with asthma who are uncontrolled. Patients and providers would be notified that a follow-up evaluation may be indicated. Criteria for being uncontrolled would include hospitalization, more than three ED visits, or more than two weeks of school missed due to asthma in the last year. These criteria could be broadened depending upon the available resources of the organization. Cross Reference(s): H3, H4, F18, F19	Feasibility of Implementation Supported by Evidence Reduce Inequalities Reduce Net Costs Improve Overall Outcomes Overall Grade Confidence in Rating
H3.	Health care delivery systems would institute electronic or other tracking mechanisms to identify patients with asthma who have not been evaluated for asthma in the past two years. Patients and providers would be notified that a follow-up evaluation may be necessary. Cross Reference(s): H2, H4, F18, F19	Feasibility of Implementation Supported by Evidence Reduce Inequalities Reduce Net Costs Improve Overall Outcomes Overall Grade Confidence in Rating
H4.	Health care systems would institute pharmacy-based tracking systems to identify patients with asthma who are uncontrolled. Uncontrolled patients are those who have received more than two bronchodilator inhalers in the past month or who have failed to refill an anti-inflammatory medication in the time expected. Automatic referrals for an outpatient evaluation would be sent to the primary asthma provider and the patient's family. Cross Reference(s): H2, H3, F18, F19	Feasibility of Implementation Supported by Evidence Reduce Inequalities Reduce Net Costs Improve Overall Outcomes Overall Grade Confidence in Rating

Improving Health Care Organization and Delivery (continued)

		Feasibility of Implementation
H5.	Federal and state governments would fund the creation of certified "asthma-provider centers" within local health care delivery system(s). The asthma center staffs would include primary and specialist providers, asthma educators, and case managers. The centers would: a) be the hub for asthma education for providers within a geographic area, b) serve as specialty asthma referral centers for children with difficult-to-control asthma and children who lack an asthma-trained health care provider, and c)assist state and local asthma surveillance units in the collection of population-based asthma surveillance data for the communities they serve.	Supported by Evidence
		Reduce Inequalities
		Reduce Net Costs
		Improve Overall Outcomes
		Overall Grade
	Cross Reference(s): F11	Confidence in Rating
H6.	National health care quality organizations would develop and monitor standards of care for asthma-related hospitalizations. These asthma hospitalization standards would include: a) a joint physician and case-manager/social worker evaluation of the reason for admission, b) the family's completion of an asthma education program before discharge, c) providing the family with a simple written plan, in the family's language, regarding actions to be taken after discharge, including a follow-up appointment within one week of discharge, and d) phone follow-up by an asthma case-manager within three weeks of discharge.	Feasibility of Implementation
		Supported by Evidence
		Reduce Inequalities
		Reduce Net Costs
		Improve Overall Outcomes
		Overall Grade
	Cross Reference(s): F10, F12	Confidence in Rating
H7.	National health care quality organizations would develop and monitor standards of care for children who have had more than three asthma-related hospitalizations in a two year period. These standards would include case-management/social work services and primary care by a certified asthma provider. Care would include an examination by the certified asthma provider at least every three months and all necessary medications and equipment ordered by that provider.	Feasibility of Implementation
		Supported by Evidence
		Reduce Inequalities
		Reduce Net Costs
		Improve Overall Outcomes
		Overall Grade
	Cross Reference(s): F7	Confidence in Rating

Improving Health Care Organization and Delivery (continued)

		Rating
H8.	National health care quality organizations, in collaboration with local asthma-surveillance units, would develop and monitor standards for the identification and evaluation of children who have survived asthma-related near death episodes. The evaluation and treatment plan for these children would include an environmental and social evaluation of the household, and monthly home visits by a health care provider for three months. These home visits would be designed to facilitate education, access to medications and equipment, compliance with medication regimens, and household environmental refurbishment.	Feasibility of Implementation Supported by Evidence Reduce Inequalities Reduce Net Costs Improve Overall Outcomes Overall Grade Confidence in Rating
	Cross Reference(s): F7	
H9.	National health care quality organizations would develop and monitor standards of care for the education and follow-up of all children discharged from the ED for asthma. These standards would include: a) providing videotape and other in-ED education and take-home written asthma instructions, b) supplying asthma medications and equipment if the family does not have them, c) making a follow-up appointment with a certified asthma provider, and d) notifying the primary provider that the child was seen in the ED for asthma.	Feasibility of Implementation Supported by Evidence Reduce Inequalities Reduce Net Costs Improve Overall Outcomes Overall Grade Confidence in Rating
	Cross Reference(s): F10, F12	
H10.	Local asthma centers, schools, and voluntary community groups would collaborate to institute a combined asthma health care and school-based program for all schools showing a high prevalence of asthma. This program would facilitate asthma education of school personnel, asthma training of school nurses, referral of children with asthma (particularly those with uncontrolled symptoms) to a local provider, availability of asthma medications and equipment in the schools, and assistance in case of emergencies.	Feasibility of Implementation Supported by Evidence Reduce Inequalities Reduce Net Costs Improve Overall Outcomes Overall Grade Confidence in Rating
	Cross Reference(s): En4, Ed4, H11, H12	
H11.	States would provide funding for all school nurses to be full time and to be trained as Certified Asthma Educators. These nurses would educate patients and other school staff and perform environmental monitoring. The nurses would be required to identify children with asthma, obtain peak flows, and develop care plans and/or appropriate referrals for those children.	Feasibility of Implementation Supported by Evidence Reduce Inequalities Reduce Net Costs Improve Overall Outcomes Overall Grade Confidence in Rating
	Cross Reference(s): Ed4, H10, H12, F15	

Improving Health Care Organization and Delivery (continued)

		Feasibility of Implementation
H12.	States would fund public health nurses trained in asthma education to cover all state certified childcare centers. These nurses would be required to identify children with asthma, obtain peak flows, and develop care plans and/or appropriate referrals for those children.	Feasibility of Implementation Supported by Evidence Reduce Inequalities Reduce Net Costs Improve Overall Outcomes Overall Grade Confidence in Rating
	Cross Reference(s): Ed4, H10, H11, F15	
H13.	Congress would create an "Asthma Peace Corps". This program would provide special training for nurses and physicians in asthma prevention and care and participants would serve as asthma educators and specialists to pay off their educational debt.	Feasibility of Implementation Supported by Evidence Reduce Inequalities Reduce Net Costs Improve Overall Outcomes Overall Grade Confidence in Rating
	Cross Reference(s): F15	

Education

Ed1.	National asthma, provider, and quality assurance organizations would set simple, minimal standards for the content of asthma education. Asthma education would be for patients/families, providers, and school personnel.	Feasibility of Implementation Supported by Evidence Reduce Inequalities Reduce Net Costs Improve Overall Outcomes Overall Grade Confidence in Rating
	Cross Reference(s): other education levers, F15, F16	
Ed2.	The U.S. Department of Health and Human Services, in collaboration with other federal and state agencies and national asthma organizations, would promote early diagnosis, referral, and treatment of patients with asthma through an educational campaign in the national media. This campaign would also target high-risk populations, such as ethnic minorities and poor individuals with uncontrolled asthma.	Feasibility of Implementation Supported by Evidence Reduce Inequalities Reduce Net Costs Improve Overall Outcomes Overall Grade Confidence in Rating

Education (continued)

		Rating
Ed3.	National sports and athletic organization(s) would undertake an educational media campaign directed at physical-education teachers, coaches, and children participating in sports activities. The campaign would use professional athletes as spokespersons and would train coaches and children to recognize asthma symptoms and the need for medication before exercise, and to administer basic emergency treatment.	Feasibility of Implementation Supported by Evidence Reduce Inequalities Reduce Net Costs Improve Overall Outcomes Overall Grade Confidence in Rating
Ed4.	National, state, and local school organizations would implement a broad-based asthma education program for teachers and children. This program would be part of the science curriculum in elementary school and high school. It would be a series of class lessons aimed at familiarizing students with the symptoms of asthma and with how to be helpful to a person with an asthma attack. The program would provide awareness of how common the condition is and how children with asthma can lead normal lives. Cross Reference(s): H10, H11, F15	Feasibility of Implementation Supported by Evidence Reduce Inequalities Reduce Net Costs Improve Overall Outcomes Overall Grade Confidence in Rating
Ed5.	Volunteer organizations with special interest and expertise in asthma (e.g., ALA, AAFA), with state and federal government support, would promote implementation of Health Department-certified asthma education and smoking-cessation programs. These organizations would work with health care organizations and schools in these implementation efforts. Cross Reference(s): En5, F15	Feasibility of Implementation Supported by Evidence Reduce Inequalities Reduce Net Costs Improve Overall Outcomes Overall Grade Confidence in Rating
Ed6.	Health care providers would provide and track the completion of a standardized basic-education course on asthma for any child newly diagnosed with asthma and his/her family. The course would include information on symptoms, how to use medications and equipment, what to do in case of an attack, and avoidance of asthma triggers. Materials for the program would be simple, interactive, in the family's language, and at the appropriate reading-level. Cross Reference(s): Ed7	Feasibility of Implementation Supported by Evidence Reduce Inequalities Reduce Net Costs Improve Overall Outcomes Overall Grade Confidence in Rating

Education (continued)

Ed7. Health care providers would provide and track the completion of an asthma education course by all families of high-risk children. High-risk children are those who have been hospitalized or in the emergency department more than three times in the last year, or have had an asthma-related life-threatening episode. Cross Reference(s): Ed6	Feasibility of Implementation Supported by Evidence Reduce Inequalities Reduce Net Costs Improve Overall Outcomes Overall Grade Confidence in Rating
Ed8. Local asthma health care centers would hold CME-like courses for all primary providers who see pediatric patients with asthma. These providers would include family-physicians, pediatricians, nurse practitioners, respiratory therapists, and pharmacists. Based on the NHLBI National Guidelines, these programs would be simplified, adapted according to the same principles as patient educational programs, and certified by the Health Department. Cross Reference(s): H5	Feasibility of Implementation Supported by Evidence Reduce Inequalities Reduce Net Costs Improve Overall Outcomes Overall Grade Confidence in Rating
Ed9. Professional pediatric and family practice associations would distribute the latest epidemiological and clinical trial data to their state and local affiliates as well as to state Medicaid associations, and HMOs. Such data would provide information on asthma prevalence and incidence, risk group profiles, and effective asthma-related therapies and interventions. Cross Reference(s): Ed10	Feasibility of Implementation Supported by Evidence Reduce Inequalities Reduce Net Costs Improve Overall Outcomes Overall Grade Confidence in Rating
Ed10. Professional associations in pediatrics and family practice, the NHLBI and other associations with an interest in asthma would mount an effort to raise asthma awareness among public policy makers. This asthma awareness campaign would target legislators and federal and state officials. Cross Reference(s): Ed9	Feasibility of Implementation Supported by Evidence Reduce Inequalities Reduce Net Costs Improve Overall Outcomes Overall Grade Confidence in Rating

Education (continued)

Ed11.	Standards for asthma education would include primary prevention education standards for pregnant women. Prenatal care providers would provide education to pregnant women regarding household risk factors for asthma (e.g. dust mites, smoke, pets, etc.) and the benefits of breastfeeding.	Feasibility of Implementation Supported by Evidence Reduce Inequalities Reduce Net Costs Improve Overall Outcomes Overall Grade Confidence in Rating
Ed12.	Health care providers would target parents of children with asthma for training as Certified Asthma Educators. These parents would then serve as local peer educators and role models.	Feasibility of Implementation Supported by Evidence Reduce Inequalities Reduce Net Costs Improve Overall Outcomes Overall Grade Confidence in Rating
	Cross Reference(s): F15	

Financing and Regulation

F1.	Private-sector and public-sector insurance programs would provide affordable health insurance for all children. Universal coverage for all children would benefit children with asthma and those who are at risk or undiagnosed. The government would provide insurance, through Medicaid, CHIP, or other means, to those children who are not eligible for other insurance programs.	Feasibility of Implementation Supported by Evidence Reduce Inequalities Reduce Net Costs Improve Overall Outcomes Overall Grade Confidence in Rating
	Cross Reference(s): F2, F3, F4, F5	
F2.	Specifically, Congress would increase the eligibility level for Medicaid to include all children in families earning up to 300 percent of the Federal poverty level. Over the course of the next decade the Medicaid eligibility level would be raised incrementally to cover increasingly larger portions of children in "working-poor" families.	Feasibility of Implementation Supported by Evidence Reduce Inequalities Reduce Net Costs Improve Overall Outcomes Overall Grade Confidence in Rating
	Cross Reference(s): F1, F3, F4, F5	

Financing and Regulation (continued)

		Feasibility of Implementation
F3.	Specifically, the Federal government would provide subsidies for employer health benefits for working families earning up to 300 percent of the Federal poverty level. This subsidy would promote health insurance coverage for "working poor" families with access to employer-based health insurance.	Supported by Evidence
		Reduce Inequalities
		Reduce Net Costs
		Improve Overall Outcomes
		Overall Grade
	Cross Reference(s): F1, F2, F4, F5	Confidence in Rating
F4.	Specifically, Congress would amend Medicaid legislation to allow for presumptive eligibility of all children. Children diagnosed with severe asthma would be eligible for immediate coverage of medical care services under the Medicaid program, regardless of the status of their eligibility paperwork.	Feasibility of Implementation
		Supported by Evidence
		Reduce Inequalities
		Reduce Net Costs
		Improve Overall Outcomes
		Overall Grade
	Cross Reference(s): F1, F2, F3, F5	Confidence in Rating
F5.	Specifically, all private and public insurance programs would provide uninterrupted health insurance coverage to all children. For example, every state Medicaid or CHIP program would adopt a 12-month continuous enrollment option so that children with asthma do not experience interrupted insurance coverage. Similar mechanisms would be put in place for private insurance to assure continued insurance coverage when a child changes insurance plans or providers.	Feasibility of Implementation
		Supported by Evidence
		Reduce Inequalities
		Reduce Net Costs
		Improve Overall Outcomes
		Overall Grade
	Cross Reference(s): F1, F2, F3, F4	Confidence in Rating
F6.	All private and public insurance programs would provide supplemental preventive benefits packages, or coordinate existing benefits, to cover all children with asthma with nominal co-payments. Preventive services covered would include age-appropriate preventive medications, equipment necessary to deliver medications, three "asthma check-up" visits with a regular provider, an initial evaluation by an interdisciplinary team, and follow-up evaluations every 5 years thereafter.	Feasibility of Implementation
		Supported by Evidence
		Reduce Inequalities
		Reduce Net Costs
		Improve Overall Outcomes
		Overall Grade
		Confidence in Rating

Financing and Regulation (continued)

F7.	All private and public insurance programs would provide supplemental extended service benefits packages to cover all children with severe asthma (e.g. hospitalized, more than three ED visits per year) with limited co-payments. Extended services covered would include all tertiary care, an environmental assessment after repeated hospitalization, an annual evaluation by an interdisciplinary team to set treatment and management goals, and case-management services to coordinate care from multiple programs and sources in order to ensure that these goals are met.	Feasibility of Implementation Supported by Evidence Reduce Inequalities Reduce Net Costs Improve Overall Outcomes Overall Grade Confidence in Rating	
F8.	Insurance programs would institute co-payment mechanisms that reward families who adhere to preventive care. For example, families would get reduced co-payments if they filled all preventive-medication prescriptions and attended all regular preventive visits.	Feasibility of Implementation Supported by Evidence Reduce Inequalities Reduce Net Costs Improve Overall Outcomes Overall Grade Confidence in Rating	
F9.	Private and public payers of care would create incentive program(s) for providers who comply with preventive care standards. For example, health providers who comply with these standards would receive financial bonuses (e.g. cash and/or extra vacation days).	Feasibility of Implementation Supported by Evidence Reduce Inequalities Reduce Net Costs Improve Overall Outcomes Overall Grade Confidence in Rating	
F10.	The appropriate national and state agencies would require that accreditation of hospitals, managed care organizations, and other providers would include evaluation of a minimum, basic set of asthma care related standards. For example, to receive NCQA accreditation, health care systems would be evaluated on their compliance with HEDIS asthma standards through site visits or random chart abstraction.	Feasibility of Implementation Supported by Evidence Reduce Inequalities Reduce Net Costs Improve Overall Outcomes Overall Grade Confidence in Rating	

Financing and Regulation (continued)

F11.	The appropriate national and state agencies would provide accreditation for "Asthma Centers of Excellence" within local health care delivery systems according to more specialized standards. To obtain "asthma certification" hospitals would demonstrate adherence to special standards such as minimum number of providers with expertise in asthma (physicians, nurse practitioners, respiratory therapists, asthma educators, and case managers) and quality assurance protocols for asthma care. Cross Reference(s): H5	Feasibility of Implementation Supported by Evidence Reduce Inequalities Reduce Net Costs Improve Overall Outcomes Overall Grade Confidence in Rating	
F12.	Private and public payers of care would require accreditation to provide basic or more specialized asthma services as part of their condition for payment for these services. For example, all managed care organizations receiving payment for asthma hospitalization and ED care would be required to meet certain minimum patient education standards prior to the patient's discharge. Cross Reference(s): H6, H7, H8, H9, F10	Feasibility of Implementation Supported by Evidence Reduce Inequalities Reduce Net Costs Improve Overall Outcomes Overall Grade Confidence in Rating	
F13.	Health departments would institute a grading scheme for health care systems and their "asthma-provider centers." The grading scheme would be based on national or state-level standards for asthma care and would promote compliance with those standards. The grading information would be provided to the public. Cross Reference(s): H5, H6, H7, H8, H9	Feasibility of Implementation Supported by Evidence Reduce Inequalities Reduce Net Costs Improve Overall Outcomes Overall Grade Confidence in Rating	
F14.	Congress and state legislators would enact legislation to penalize payers of care who selectively disenroll children who have high utilization of services, unless the disenrollment is for the purpose of transferring the patient to coverage under the SSI program. Some children with asthma are hospitalized and use the ED multiple times because of the baseline severity of their illness. Payers would be held accountable for financial and other costs to the child with asthma and his/her family as a result of the disenrollment.	Feasibility of Implementation Supported by Evidence Reduce Inequalities Reduce Net Costs Improve Overall Outcomes Overall Grade Confidence in Rating	

Financing and Regulation (continued)

		Rating
F15.	States would develop mechanisms for certification of asthma educators following national standards. For example, certification would be granted through examination or documentation of prior specialist training, or extended working experience with this population. Any health provider or allied health professional (e.g., health educators, social workers, case managers, respiratory therapists) may be eligible for this certification. A state board designated by the state health department would oversee the certification process and its implementation, including possible linkage of asthma education certification to reimbursement level of services. Cross Reference(s): Ed4, Ed12, H10, H11, H12, H13, F16	Feasibility of Implementation Supported by Evidence Reduce Inequalities Reduce Net Costs Improve Overall Outcomes Overall Grade Confidence in Rating
F16.	The American Boards of Pediatrics, Family Medicine, and other primary child health care providers would institute an asthma-specific core module in their national certification process for all their diplomates. These modules would include asthma diagnosis, evaluation of symptom control, indication for anti-inflammatory therapy, and key elements regarding patient education (e.g., medication and equipment use and avoidance of asthma triggers.) Diplomates who by examination score above a certain threshold would receive an asthma certificate that would qualify them as a certified asthma educator and experienced provider. Cross Reference(s): Ed8, F15, F17	Feasibility of Implementation Supported by Evidence Reduce Inequalities Reduce Net Costs Improve Overall Outcomes Overall Grade Confidence in Rating
F17.	Accreditation bodies would require that all managed care organizations or integrated health care systems providing care for children with asthma have providers "experienced" in pediatric asthma in their networks. For instance, documentation of at least one annual visit with an "experienced provider" or in consultation with an "experienced provider" would be required for all children with asthma. Cross Reference(s): F16	Feasibility of Implementation Supported by Evidence Reduce Inequalities Reduce Net Costs Improve Overall Outcomes Overall Grade Confidence in Rating
F18.	Public and private purchasers of health care would evaluate claims for pediatric asthma cases to monitor quality of care. In areas where asthma is a reportable condition, health care payers and surveillance units would link their data systems to measure timing and adequacy of care. Results of these evaluations would be used to reward and/or sanction plans/providers. Cross Reference(s): P1, F9, F10, F12, F13, F14, F19	Feasibility of Implementation Supported by Evidence Reduce Inequalities Reduce Net Costs Improve Overall Outcomes Overall Grade Confidence in Rating

Financing and Regulation (continued)

F19.	Accreditation bodies would require hospitals and managed care organizations to establish information systems to track and report on pediatric asthma patients or to have such systems ready within three years. Cross Reference(s): H2, H3, H4, F10, F13, F18		Feasibility of Implementation Supported by Evidence Reduce Inequalities Reduce Net Costs Improve Overall Outcomes Overall Grade Confidence in Rating

Other

O1.	The Department of Health and Human Services, in collaboration with other Federal and state health, environmental and housing agencies, would develop and implement a broad national asthma prevention research agenda. Research funding would be provided by the appropriate Federal agencies to investigate the feasibility and effectiveness of primary, secondary and tertiary community based asthma prevention programs. Cross Reference(s): O2, O3		Feasibility of Implementation Supported by Evidence Reduce Inequalities Reduce Net Costs Improve Overall Outcomes Overall Grade Confidence in Rating
O2.	Specifically, the Federal government would provide funding for research on the feasibility and cost-effectiveness of asthma screening. This research would focus on: a) the development and evaluation of reliable and valid asthma screening tools b) the impact of screening on asthma treatment and outcomes and c) the feasibility of asthma screening in schools and as part of well-child health care visits. Cross Reference(s): O1, O3		Feasibility of Implementation Supported by Evidence Reduce Inequalities Reduce Net Costs Improve Overall Outcomes Overall Grade Confidence in Rating
O3.	Specifically, public and private organizations would fund prospective research to evaluate the effect of intensive in-utero and early-life home environmental control (e.g. smoking cessation and elimination of mite and cockroach-infested areas) in preventing asthma in children at risk. Children at risk would include those who have a family history of asthma, were premature, or wheezed in the first year of life. Cross Reference(s): O1, O2		Feasibility of Implementation Supported by Evidence Reduce Inequalities Reduce Net Costs Improve Overall Outcomes Overall Grade Confidence in Rating

Appendix F
Description of Committee Ratings

This spreadsheet shows the analysis of the ratings provided by the committee members for the 63 levers. In this analysis, we use average ratings to summarize a lever, where the average is taken across all committee members. Generally, all eleven members responded to each question, but if not, we take the average across all individuals who responded.

The first statistic we calculated for each lever is its average overall grade. This statistic is shown in the sixth column. For example, the first row of data contains information on lever O1 (the lever ID is shown in the second column). This lever's average overall grade is 3.6, which is the average overall grade across the 6 members who voted an "A" (score of 4); and the 4 committee members who voted a "B" (score of 3) $(((6*4)+(4*3))/10=3.6)$. One member did not respond and does not affect the average.

Note that the levers have been sorted from highest to lowest in terms of overall grade, with lever O1 receiving the highest average grade of all 63 levers rated. Thus, this lever has the highest rank of "1," shown in the first column. Note that the ranks go from best or highest average overall grade ("1") to worst or lowest average overall grade ("63"). Ties are shown in a specific manner. For example, levers H1 and F5 are tied, and thus are given ranks "5a" and "5b" respectively (H1 preceded F5 in the original list of levers, so it received the "5a" ranking).

We continue with our discussion of lever O1. We skip columns 3, 4, and 5 for the moment. In the sixth column, the average overall grade is shown for this lever: 3.6. This grade is ranked 1st (the seventh column) among all average overall grades. It should be first, as the rows are sorted by this statistic. The rank in the seventh column is similar to that shown in the first column, except if there are ties, the latter appends an "a," "b," etc. as appropriate.

At the top of the page over columns 6 and 7, one sees the distribution statistics for the average overall grades across all levers: the min was 1.9, the 25th percentile was 2.5, the median was 2.8, the 75th percentile was 3.0, and the max was 3.6. The mean is also given (2.8) as well as the standard deviation (0.4).

The next column (the eighth) shows the answer to the question "was this lever in the top 20 levers in terms of average overall grade?" Due to the sorting of levers by average overall grade, one sees a "YES" in this column for the first 20 levers. At the top of this column one sees the total number of levers that answer "yes" to this question, 20 levers must be in the top 20, so the total is 20.

Let's skip columns 9 and 10 for the moment.

The next 3 columns (11-13) show the results for the feasibility criterion. The statistic for each lever is the feasibility score averaged across all committee members who answered that question. So for lever O1, the average feasibility score was 3.4. This feasibility score was the 4th highest across all levers, as shown in the rank column. One also sees the distribution statistics for the feasibility scores at the top of the feasibility columns. The last column in this group has the answer to the question "did this lever score in the top 67% of the average feasibility scores?" What this translates into, given that we have 63 levers, is whether the rank of the feasibility score is 42 or lower.

We then display similar groups of columns for the evidence, inequalities, costs, outcomes, and confidence criteria.

The last column on the page shows the percent of all scores missing for a lever. Note that 11 members were each asked 7 questions per lever (overall grade plus the six criteria of feasibility through confidence), so a lever had to have 77 answers to have complete data or 0% missing data. So for lever O1, 9% of the 77 answers were missing. Note that this means 9% of the total 77 answers (or 7 answers) were missing. Perhaps all seven answers were associated with one individual, or perhaps seven different committee members missed one answer each. This 9% does not mean that 9% of the 11 members missed at least one answer.

Now go back to columns 9 and 10. In column 9, the answer to the question "did this lever score in the top 67% of the scores for all five dimensions feasibility, evidence, inequalities, costs, and outcomes?" We can see for lever O1 the answer is YES, as we see Y's all across the row under each dimension. Note that the confidence criterion is not included in this summary statistic. Note also that at the top of column 9 we can see the total number of levers that answered YES (21 levers did) in column 9.

In column 10 we ask the question "did the lever have an average overall grade in the top 20, AND did it score in the top 67% of the score for all 5 dimensions?" For a lever to have a "YES" to this question, it needs a "Y" in both columns 8 and 9. Lever O1 does so and in total 17 levers do. Such a lever is denoted as "IN" and its row is in gray scale; otherwise the lever is denoted "OUT."

We now return to the third through fifth columns. In the third column, we state the summary decision of "IN" or "OUT" for easy reference. Column 4 gives the lever statement. The fifth column "References" shows those levers that should be considered related to lever O1. In addition to the names of the levers (O2 and O3), we give their ranks and final decisions of "IN" or "OUT." Lever O2 is ranked 26c and is "OUT," and lever O3 is ranked 35c and is "OUT."

Consider the second row, containing information on lever F1. It scores second in terms of average overall grade at 3.4; however, it does not satisfy all 5 dimensions - this is why one sees a "Y, N, N" in columns 8, 9 and 10. Where do the no's come from? This lever scores below the 67th percentile in terms of feasibility at 2.3. In fact, it is ranked 54th on this dimension. As a result, this lever is "OUT" and is not in gray scale.

Rank	Lever ID	IN or OUT	Lever	References	Overall grade (averaged over all members) min / 25th / median / 75th / max / mean / sd	Overall grade	Rank	In top 20 levers in terms of overall grade?	hidden for summing	In top 67% for all five dimensions (a)-(e)?	hidden for summing	Satisfy both grade and dimension criteria?	hidden for summing	Feasibility (averaged) min / 25th / median / 75th / max / mean / sd	Feasibility	Rank	In top 67% in terms of feasibility?	Evidence (averaged) min / 25th / median / 75th / max / mean / sd	Evidence	Rank	In top 67% in terms of evidence?	Inequalities (averaged) min / 25th / median / 75th / max / mean / sd	Inequalities	Rank	In top 67% in terms of inequalities?	Costs (averaged) min / 25th / median / 75th / max / mean / sd	Costs	Rank	In top 67% in terms of costs?	Outcomes (averaged) min / 25th / median / 75th / max / mean / sd	Outcomes	Rank	In top 67% in terms of outcomes?	Confidence (averaged) min / 25th / median / 75th / max / mean / sd	Confidence	Rank	In top 67% in terms of confidence?	% missing scores across all members and all criteria
1	O1	IN	The Department of Health and Human Services, in collaboration with other Federal and state health, environmental and housing agencies, would develop and implement a broad national asthma prevention research agenda. Research funding would be provided by the appropriate Federal agencies to investigate the feasibility and effectiveness of primary, secondary and tertiary community based asthma prevention programs.	O2 (26c, OUT) O3 (35c, OUT)	1.9 / 2.5 / 2.8 / 3.0 / 3.6 / 2.8 / 0.4	3.6	1	Y	1	Y	1	Y	1	1.7 / 2.5 / 2.7 / 3.1 / 3.6 / 2.7 / 0.4	3.4	4	Y	1.6 / 2.3 / 2.6 / 2.9 / 3.4 / 2.6 / 0.4	3.3	2	Y	2.0 / 2.5 / 2.8 / 3.0 / 3.8 / 2.8 / 0.4	3.4	6	Y	2.0 / 2.3 / 2.5 / 2.7 / 3.1 / 2.5 / 0.3	2.9	3	Y	2.0 / 2.5 / 2.7 / 2.9 / 3.5 / 2.7 / 0.3	3.2	4	Y	2.5 / 3.0 / 3.1 / 3.2 / 3.5 / 3.1 / 0.2	3.5	1	Y	9%
2	F1	OUT	Private-sector and public-sector insurance programs would provide affordable health insurance for all children. Universal coverage for all children would benefit children with asthma and those who are at risk or undiagnosed. The government would provide insurance, through Medicaid, CHIP, or other means, to those children who are not eligible for other insurance programs.	F2 (7b, IN) F3 (26b, OUT) F4 (33, OUT) F5 (5b, IN)		3.4	2	Y	1	N	0	N	0		2.3	54	N		3.3	4	Y		3.8	1	Y		2.5	23	Y		3.5	1	Y		3.5	1	Y	3%

Legend of benchmark statistics (per dimension, "averaged over all members"):

Statistic	Overall grade	Feasibility	Evidence	Inequalities	Costs	Outcomes	Confidence
min	1.9	1.7	1.6	2.0	2.0	2.0	2.5
25th	2.5	2.5	2.3	2.5	2.3	2.5	3.0
median	2.8	2.7	2.6	2.8	2.5	2.7	3.1
75th	3.0	3.1	2.9	3.0	2.7	2.9	3.2
max	3.6	3.6	3.4	3.8	3.1	3.5	3.5
mean	2.8	2.7	2.6	2.8	2.5	2.7	3.1
sd	0.4	0.4	0.4	0.4	0.3	0.3	0.2

Summary column totals: In top 20 levers in terms of overall grade? (Total = 20); In top 67% for all five dimensions (a)-(e)? (Total = 21); Satisfy both grade and dimension criteria? (Total = 17)

Lever data:

Rank	Lever ID	IN or OUT	Lever	References	Overall grade	Overall Rank	In top 20 levers in terms of overall grade?	hidden for summing	In top 67% for all five dimensions (a)-(e)?	hidden for summing	Satisfy both grade and dimension criteria?	hidden for summing	Feasibility	Feas. Rank	In top 67% in terms of feasibility?	Evidence	Evid. Rank	In top 67% in terms of evidence?	Inequalities	Ineq. Rank	In top 67% in terms of inequalities?	Costs	Cost Rank	In top 67% in terms of costs?	Outcomes	Out. Rank	In top 67% in terms of outcomes?	Confidence	Conf. Rank	In top 67% in terms of confidence?	% missing scores across all members and all criteria
3	Ed2	IN	The U.S. Department of Health and Human Services, in collaboration with other federal and state agencies and national asthma organizations, would promote early diagnosis, referral, and treatment of patients with asthma through an educational campaign in the national media. This campaign would also target high-risk populations, such as ethnic minorities and poor individuals with uncontrolled asthma.		3.3	3	Y	1	Y	1	Y	1	3.2	9	Y	2.6	33	Y	3.1	12	Y	2.7	17	Y	2.8	28	Y	3.0	40	Y	16%
4	Ed7	IN	Health care providers would provide and track the completion of an asthma education course by all families of high-risk children. High-risk children are those who have been hospitalized or in the emergency department more than three times in the last year, or have had an asthma-related life-threatening episode.	Ed6 (13b, IN)	3.3	4	Y	1	Y	1	Y	1	2.9	23	Y	3.1	7	Y	2.9	19	Y	2.9	3	Y	3.0	10	Y	3.1	35	Y	6%

Summary statistics (averaged over all members), reference values:

Statistic	Overall grade	Feasibility	Evidence	Inequalities	Costs	Outcomes	Confidence
min	1.9	1.7	1.6	2.0	2.0	2.0	2.5
25th	2.5	2.5	2.3	2.5	2.3	2.5	3.0
median	2.8	2.7	2.6	2.8	2.5	2.7	3.1
75th	3.0	3.1	2.9	3.0	2.7	2.9	3.2
max	3.6	3.6	3.4	3.8	3.1	3.5	3.5
mean	2.8	2.7	2.6	2.8	2.5	2.7	3.1
sd	0.4	0.4	0.4	0.4	0.3	0.3	0.2

Lever data:

Rank	Lever ID	IN or OUT	Lever	References	Overall grade	Overall grade Rank	In top 20 levers in terms of overall grade?	(hidden for summing)	In top 67% for all five dimensions (a)-(e)?	(hidden for summing)	Satisfy both grade and dimension criteria?	(hidden for summing)	Feasibility	Feasibility Rank	In top 67% in terms of feasibility?	Evidence	Evidence Rank	In top 67% in terms of evidence?	Inequalities	Inequalities Rank	In top 67% in terms of inequalities?	Costs	Costs Rank	In top 67% in terms of costs?	Outcomes	Outcomes Rank	In top 67% in terms of outcomes?	Confidence	Confidence Rank	In top 67% in terms of confidence?	% missing scores across all members and all criteria
							Total		Total		Total			Rank			Rank			Rank		Costs	Rank		Out-comes	Rank		Confi-dence	Rank		
5a	H1	IN	Health care systems would institute quality-improvement strategies to assess and improve the quality of asthma care in different settings, according to national quality-of-care standards. Quality improvement strategies would include standardized forms, clinical protocols, and audit and feedback mechanisms. The different settings would be EDs, hospitals, and outpatient clinics.		3.3	5	Y (20)	1	Y (21)	1	Y (17)	1	2.8	26	Y	3.3	4	Y	3.1	15	Y	3.1	1	Y	3.3	2	Y	3.5	4	Y	0%
5b	F5	IN	Specifically, all private and public insurance programs would provide uninterrupted health insurance coverage to all children. For example, every state Medicaid or CHIP program would adopt a 12-month continuous enrollment option so that children with asthma do not experience interrupted insurance coverage. Similar mechanisms would be put in place for private insurance to assure continued insurance coverage when a child changes insurance plans or providers.	F1 (2, OUT) F2 (7b, IN) F3 (26b, OUT) F4 (33, OUT)	3.3	5	Y	1	Y	1	Y	1	3.0	19	Y	3.1	7	Y	3.5	5	Y	2.7	12	Y	3.3	2	Y	3.5	4	Y	1%

Rank	Lever ID	IN or OUT	Lever	References	Overall grade	Rank	In top 20 levers in terms of overall grade? (Total)	hidden for summing	In top 67% for all five dimensions (a)-(e)? (Total)	hidden for summing	Satisfy both grade and dimension criteria? (Total)	hidden for summing	Feasibility	Rank	In top 67% in terms of feasibility?	Evidence	Rank	In top 67% in terms of evidence?	Inequalities	Rank	In top 67% in terms of inequalities?	Costs	Rank	In top 67% in terms of costs?	Outcomes	Rank	In top 67% in terms of outcomes?	Confidence	Rank	In top 67% in terms of confidence?	% missing scores across all members and all criteria
					min 1.9 / 25th 2.5 / median 2.8 / 75th 3.0 / max 3.6 / mean 2.8 / sd 0.4								min 1.7 / 25th 2.5 / median 2.7 / 75th 3.1 / max 3.6 / mean 2.7 / sd 0.4			min 1.6 / 25th 2.3 / median 2.6 / 75th 2.9 / max 3.4 / mean 2.6 / sd 0.4			min 2.0 / 25th 2.5 / median 2.8 / 75th 3.0 / max 3.8 / mean 2.8 / sd 0.4			min 2.0 / 25th 2.3 / median 2.5 / 75th 2.7 / max 3.1 / mean 2.5 / sd 0.3			min 2.0 / 25th 2.5 / median 2.7 / 75th 2.9 / max 3.5 / mean 2.7 / sd 0.3			min 2.5 / 25th 3.0 / median 3.1 / 75th 3.2 / max 3.5 / mean 3.1 / sd 0.2			
7a	P4	IN	State health departments, working with local asthma-surveillance units, would conduct more detailed surveillance of those subgroups or geographic areas that have worse outcomes. Surveillance would include a survey of risk factors that are both amenable to interventions and that have been shown in recent research to be associated with asthma-related outcomes.		3.2	7	Y (20)	1	Y (21)	1	Y (17)	1	3.3	6	Y	3.0	11	Y	3.5	3	Y	2.8	10	Y	2.7	35	Y	3.2	16	Y	9%
7b	F2	IN	Specifically, Congress would increase the eligibility level for Medicaid to include all children in families earning up to 300 percent of the Federal poverty level. Over the course of the next decade the Medicaid eligibility level would be raised incrementally to cover increasingly larger portions of children in "working-poor" families.	F1 (2, OUT) F3 (26b, OUT) F4 (33, OUT) F5 (5b, IN)	3.2	7	Y	1	Y	1	Y	1	2.5	40	Y	2.8	19	Y	3.8	1	Y	2.5	23	Y	3.2	5	Y	3.4	7	Y	1%

Rank	Lever ID	IN or OUT	Lever	References	Overall grade	Rank	In top 20 levers in terms of overall grade?	hidden for summing	In top 67% for all five dimensions (a)-(e)?	hidden for summing	Satisfy both grade and dimension criteria?	hidden for summing	Feasibility	Rank	In top 67% in terms of feasibility?	Evidence	Rank	In top 67% in terms of evidence?	Inequalities	Rank	In top 67% in terms of inequalities?	Costs	Rank	In top 67% in terms of costs?	Outcomes	Rank	In top 67% in terms of outcomes?	Confidence	Rank	In top 67% in terms of confidence?	% missing scores across all members and all criteria
					min 1.9 / 25th 2.5 / median 2.8 / 75th 3.0 / max 3.6 / mean 2.8 / sd 0.4		Total		Total		Total		min 1.7 / 25th 2.5 / median 2.7 / 75th 3.1 / max 3.6 / mean 2.7 / sd 0.4			min 1.6 / 25th 2.3 / median 2.6 / 75th 2.9 / max 3.4 / mean 2.6 / sd 0.4			min 2.0 / 25th 2.5 / median 2.8 / 75th 3.0 / max 3.8 / mean 2.8 / sd 0.4			min 2.0 / 25th 2.3 / median 2.5 / 75th 2.7 / max 3.1 / mean 2.5 / sd 0.3			min 2.0 / 25th 2.5 / median 2.7 / 75th 2.9 / max 3.5 / mean 2.7 / sd 0.3			min 2.5 / 25th 3.0 / median 3.1 / 75th 3.2 / max 3.5 / mean 3.1 / sd 0.2			
					Overall grade	Rank	20		21		17		Feasibility	Rank		Evidence	Rank		Inequalities	Rank		Costs	Rank		Outcomes	Rank		Confidence	Rank		
9a	P3	IN	The Centers for Disease Control and Prevention, acting as lead agency within the U.S. Department of Health and Human Services, and in collaboration with other federal and state agencies, would refine their standards for asthma-surveillance data. These standards would include: a) asthma-related "sentinel events" (e.g. hospitalizations, near death events) to be collected from public health agencies and health care organizations and b) other asthma severity indicators to identify high-risk populations.		3.2	9	Y	1	Y	1	Y	1	3.6	1	Y	3.1	9	Y	2.8	27	Y	2.5	31	Y	2.7	32	Y	3.2	21	Y	0%
9b	En5	IN	States would enact legislation to use tobacco taxes and legal settlements to fund the creation and operation of a free, Health Department-certified smoking-cessation program. Health care providers and school personnel would refer all smoking persons who live in a household with a child with asthma or who work in a school.		3.2	9	Y	1	Y	1	Y	1	3.1	14	Y	3.3	4	Y	2.9	19	Y	2.8	5	Y	3.1	8	Y	3.3	14	Y	1%

Rank	Lever ID	IN or OUT	Lever	References	Overall grade averaged over all members							Overall grade	Rank	In top 20 levers in terms of overall grade? Total	hidden for summing	In top 67% for all five dimensions (a)-(e)? Total	hidden for summing	Satisfy both grade and dimension criteria? Total	hidden for summing	Feasibility averaged over all members							Feasibility	Rank	In top 67% in terms of feasibility?	Evidence averaged over all members							Evidence	Rank	In top 67% in terms of evidence?	Inequalities averaged over all members							Inequalities	Rank	In top 67% in terms of inequalities?	Costs averaged over all members							Costs	Rank	In top 67% in terms of costs?	Outcomes averaged over all members							Outcomes	Rank	In top 67% in terms of outcomes?	Confidence averaged over all members							Confidence	Rank	In top 67% in terms of confidence?	% missing scores across all members and all criteria
					min	25th	median	75th	max	mean	sd												min	25th	median	75th	max	mean	sd				min	25th	median	75th	max	mean	sd				min	25th	median	75th	max	mean	sd				min	25th	median	75th	max	mean	sd				min	25th	median	75th	max	mean	sd				min	25th	median	75th	max	mean	sd				
					1.9	2.5	2.8	3.0	3.6	2.8	0.4												1.7	2.5	2.7	3.1	3.6	2.7	0.4				1.6	2.3	2.6	2.9	3.4	2.6	0.4				2.0	2.5	2.8	3.0	3.8	2.8	0.4				2.0	2.3	2.5	2.7	3.1	2.5	0.3				2.0	2.5	2.7	2.9	3.5	2.7	0.3				2.5	3.0	3.1	3.2	3.5	3.1	0.2				
9c	Eng8	IN	Public and private payers of care would extend durable medical equipment coverage to items proven to reduce the exacerbations of asthma. Such items would include mattresses, pillow covers and other items that play an important role in preventing exposure to known allergens.	Other financing and regulation levers								3.2	9	Y 20	1	Y 21	1	Y 17	1								3.0	19	Y								3.4	1	Y								3.3	8	Y								2.8	5	Y								2.8	20	Y								3.4	7	Y	0%
12	H4	IN	Health care systems would institute pharmacy-based tracking systems to identify patients with asthma who are uncontrolled. Uncontrolled patients are those who have received more than two bronchodilator inhalers in the past month or who have failed to refill an anti-inflammatory medication in the time expected. Automatic referrals for an outpatient evaluation would be sent to the primary asthma provider and the patient's family.	H2 (15a, IN) H3 (54b, OUT) F18 (61, OUT) F19 (58, OUT)								3.1	12	Y	1	Y	1	Y	1								3.3	8	Y								2.6	27	Y								2.7	37	Y								2.6	19	Y								2.8	20	Y								3.2	21	Y	3%

					Overall grade averaged over all members		In top 20 levers in terms of overall grade?	hidden for summing	In top 67% for all five dimensions (a)-(e)?	hidden for summing	Satisfy both grade and dimension criteria?	hidden for summing	Feasibility averaged over all members		In top 67% in terms of feasibility?	Evidence averaged over all members		In top 67% in terms of evidence?	Inequalities averaged over all members		In top 67% in terms of inequalities?	Costs averaged over all members		In top 67% in terms of costs?	Outcomes averaged over all members		In top 67% in terms of outcomes?	Confidence averaged over all members		In top 67% in terms of confidence?	% missing scores across all members and all criteria
					min	1.9							min	1.7		min	1.6		min	2.0		min	2.0		min	2.0		min	2.5		
					25th	2.5							25th	2.5		25th	2.3		25th	2.5		25th	2.3		25th	2.5		25th	3.0		
					median	2.8							median	2.7		median	2.6		median	2.8		medi-an	2.5		median	2.7		median	3.1		
					75th	3.0							75th	3.1		75th	2.9		75th	3.0		75th	2.7		75th	2.9		75th	3.2		
					max	3.6							max	3.6		max	3.4		max	3.8		max	3.1		max	3.5		max	3.5		
					mean	2.8							mean	2.7		mean	2.6		mean	2.8		mean	2.5		mean	2.7		mean	3.1		
					sd	0.4	Total		Total		Total		sd	0.4		sd	0.4		sd	0.4		sd	0.3		sd	0.3		sd	0.2		
Rank	Lever ID	IN or OUT	Lever	Refer-ences	Overall grade	Rank	20		21		17		Feasibility	Rank		Evidence	Rank		Inequali-ties	Rank		Costs	Rank		Out-comes	Rank		Confi-dence	Rank		
13a	Ed3	IN	National sports and athletic organization(s) would undertake an educational media campaign directed at physical-education teachers, coaches, and children participating in sports activities. The campaign would use professional athletes as spokespersons and would train coaches and children to recognize asthma symptoms and the need for medication before exercise, and to administer basic emergency treatment.		3.1	13	Y	1	Y	1	Y	1	3.1	14	Y	2.6	30	Y	2.9	26	Y	2.6	21	Y	2.8	28	Y	2.7	60	N	10%
13b	Ed6	IN	Health care providers would provide and track the completion of a standardized basic-education course on asthma for any child newly diagnosed with asthma and his/her family. The course would include information on symptoms, how to use medications and equipment, what to do in case of an attack, and avoidance of asthma triggers. Materials for the program would be simple, interactive, in the family's language, and at the appropriate reading-level.	Ed7 (4, IN)	3.1	13	Y	1	Y	1	Y	1	2.8	26	Y	3.0	11	Y	2.8	32	Y	2.7	14	Y	2.9	15	Y	3.0	40	Y	6%

Rank	Lever ID	IN or OUT	Lever	References	Overall grade	Rank	In top 20 levers in terms of overall grade?	hidden for summing	In top 67% for all five dimensions (a)-(e)?	hidden for summing	Satisfy both grade and dimension criteria?	hidden for summing	Feasibility	Rank	In top 67% in terms of feasibility?	Evidence	Rank	In top 67% in terms of evidence?	Inequalities	Rank	In top 67% in terms of inequalities?	Costs	Rank	In top 67% in terms of costs?	Outcomes	Rank	In top 67% in terms of outcomes?	Confidence	Rank	In top 67% in terms of confidence?	% missing scores across all members and all criteria
(stat legend)					min 1.9 / 25th 2.5 / median 2.8 / 75th 3.0 / max 3.6 / mean 2.8 / sd 0.4							Total	min 1.7 / 25th 2.5 / median 2.7 / 75th 3.1 / max 3.6 / mean 2.7 / sd 0.4			min 1.6 / 25th 2.3 / median 2.6 / 75th 2.9 / max 3.4 / mean 2.6 / sd 0.4			min 2.0 / 25th 2.5 / median 2.8 / 75th 3.0 / max 3.8 / mean 2.8 / sd 0.4			min 2.0 / 25th 2.3 / median 2.5 / 75th 2.7 / max 3.1 / mean 2.5 / sd 0.3			min 2.0 / 25th 2.5 / median 2.7 / 75th 2.9 / max 3.5 / mean 2.7 / sd 0.3			min 2.5 / 25th 3.0 / median 3.1 / 75th 3.2 / max 3.5 / mean 3.1 / sd 0.2			
15a	H2	IN	Health care delivery systems would institute electronic or other tracking mechanisms to identify patients with asthma who are uncontrolled. Patients and providers would be notified that a follow-up evaluation may be indicated. Criteria for being uncontrolled would include hospitalization, more than three ED visits, or more than two weeks of school missed due to asthma in the last year. These criteria could be broadened depending upon the available resources of the organization.	H3 (54b, OUT), H4 (12, IN), F18 (61, OUT), F19 (58, OUT)	3.1	15	Y	1	Y	1	Y	1	2.7	31	Y	3.1	9	Y	2.8	27	Y	2.8	5	Y	3.0	10	Y	3.4	7	Y	0%
(totals for 15a)						15	20		21		17																				
15b	F10	OUT	The appropriate national and state agencies would require that accreditation of hospitals, managed care organizations, and other providers would include evaluation of a minimum, basic set of asthma care related standards. For example, to receive NCQA accreditation, health care systems would be evaluated on their compliance with HEDIS asthma standards through site visits or random chart abstraction.		3.1	15	Y	1	N	0	N	0	3.1	14	Y	2.5	34	Y	2.5	47	N	2.5	23	Y	2.8	20	Y	2.9	51	N	1%

	Rank	17a
	Lever ID	H9
	IN or OUT	OUT
	Lever	National health care quality organizations would develop and monitor standards of care for the education and follow-up of all children discharged from the ED for asthma. These standards would include: a) providing videotape and other in-ED education and take-home written asthma instructions, b) supplying asthma medications and equipment if the family does not have them, c) making a follow-up appointment with a certified asthma provider, and d) notifying the primary provider that the child was seen in the ED for asthma.
	References	F10 (15b, OUT) F12 (43f, OUT)

Overall grade averaged over all members

min	1.9
25th	2.5
median	2.8
75th	3.0
max	3.6
mean	2.8
sd	0.4
Overall grade	3.0
Rank	17
In top 20 levers in terms of overall grade? (Total 20)	Y
hidden for summing	1
In top 67% for all five dimensions (a)-(e)? (Total 21)	N
hidden for summing	0
Satisfy both grade and dimension criteria? (Total 17)	N
hidden for summing	0

Feasibility averaged over all members

min	1.7
25th	2.5
median	2.7
75th	3.1
max	3.6
mean	2.7
sd	0.4
Feasibility	2.9
Rank	23
In top 67% in terms of feasibility?	Y

Evidence averaged over all members

min	1.6
25th	2.3
median	2.6
75th	2.9
max	3.4
mean	2.6
sd	0.4
Evidence	2.4
Rank	45
In top 67% in terms of evidence?	N

Inequalities averaged over all members

Stat	Value
min	2.0
25th	2.5
median	2.8
75th	3.0
max	3.8
mean	2.8
sd	0.4
Inequalities	2.9
Rank	19
In top 67% in terms of inequalities?	Y

Costs averaged over all members

Stat	Value
min	2.0
25th	2.3
median	2.5
75th	2.7
max	3.1
mean	2.5
sd	0.3
Costs	2.6
Rank	19
In top 67% in terms of costs?	Y

Outcomes averaged over all members

Stat	Value
min	2.0
25th	2.5
median	2.7
75th	2.9
max	3.5
mean	2.7
sd	0.3
Outcomes	2.8
Rank	25
In top 67% in terms of outcomes?	Y

Confidence averaged over all members

min	2.5
25th	3.0
median	3.1
75th	3.2
max	3.5
mean	3.1
sd	0.2
Confidence	3.1
Rank	30
In top 67% in terms of confidence?	Y
% missing scores across all members and all criteria	5%

Rank	Lever ID	IN or OUT	Lever	References	Overall grade	Overall grade Rank	In top 20 levers in terms of overall grade?	hidden for summing	In top 67% for all five dimensions (a)-(e)?	hidden for summing	Satisfy both grade and dimension criteria?	hidden for summing	Feasibility	Feasibility Rank	In top 67% in terms of feasibility?	Evidence	Evidence Rank	In top 67% in terms of evidence?	Inequalities	Inequalities Rank	In top 67% in terms of inequalities?	Costs	Costs Rank	In top 67% in terms of costs?	Outcomes	Outcomes Rank	In top 67% in terms of outcomes?	Confidence	Confidence Rank	In top 67% in terms of confidence?	% missing scores across all members and all criteria
					Total 20			Total 21		Total 17																					
17b	H10	IN	Local asthma centers, schools, and voluntary community groups would collaborate to institute a combined asthma health care and school-based program for all schools showing a high prevalence of asthma. This program would facilitate asthma education of school personnel, asthma training of school nurses, referral of children with asthma (particularly those with uncontrolled symptoms) to a local provider, availability of asthma medications and equipment in the schools, and assistance in case of emergencies.	En4 (43b, OUT) Bd4 (21e, OUT) H11 (35a, H12 (43c, OUT)	3.0	17	Y	1	Y	1	Y	1	3.0	19	Y	2.9	16	Y	3.4	7	Y	3.0	2	Y	3.2	5	Y	3.4	7	Y	0%
17c	Ed1	IN	National asthma, provider, and quality assurance organizations would set simple, minimal standards for the content of asthma education. Asthma education would be for patients/families, providers, and school personnel.	Other education levers; F15 (54d, OUT) F16 (29, OUT)	3.0	17	Y	1	Y	1	Y	1	3.4	4	Y	3.0	11	Y	2.8	35	Y	2.4	35	Y	2.7	39	Y	2.9	55	N	16%

Column statistics (averaged over all members):

Statistic	Overall grade	Feasibility	Evidence	Inequalities	Costs	Outcomes	Confidence
min	1.9	1.7	1.6	2.0	2.0	2.0	2.5
25th	2.5	2.5	2.3	2.5	2.3	2.5	3.0
median	2.8	2.7	2.6	2.8	2.5	2.7	3.1
75th	3.0	3.1	2.9	3.0	2.7	2.9	3.2
max	3.6	3.6	3.4	3.8	3.1	3.5	3.5
mean	2.8	2.7	2.6	2.8	2.5	2.7	3.1
sd	0.4	0.4	0.4	0.4	0.3	0.3	0.2

Field	Ed5 (Rank 17d)	P1 (Rank 21a)
Lever ID	Ed5	P1
IN or OUT	IN	OUT
Lever	Volunteer organizations with special interest and expertise in asthma (e.g., ALA, AAFA), with state and federal government support, would promote implementation of Health Department-certified asthma education and smoking-cessation programs. These organizations would work with health care organizations and schools in these implementation efforts.	Congress and states would enact legislation to fund the creation and operation of asthma-surveillance units at the state and local level. These units would: a) collect and summarize asthma-specific data from health care organizations (e.g. asthma hospitalizations) and ongoing population-based surveys (e.g. NHIS) and b) coordinate data transfer to public and private parties for use in research and service delivery programs aimed at improving asthma care and outcomes.
References	En5 (9b, IN) F15 (54d, OUT)	F18 (61, OUT)
Overall grade — min	1.9	
Overall grade — 25th	2.5	
Overall grade — median	2.8	
Overall grade — 75th	3.0	
Overall grade — max	3.6	
Overall grade — mean	2.8	
Overall grade — sd	0.4	
Overall grade	3.0	2.9
Rank	17	21
In top 20 levers in terms of overall grade? (Total)	20 — Y	N
hidden for summing	1	0
In top 67% for all five dimensions (a)-(e)? (Total)	21 — Y	N
hidden for summing	1	0
Satisfy both grade and dimension criteria? (Total)	17 — Y	N
hidden for summing	1	0
Feasibility — min	1.7	
Feasibility — 25th	2.5	
Feasibility — median	2.7	
Feasibility — 75th	3.1	
Feasibility — max	3.6	
Feasibility — mean	2.7	
Feasibility — sd	0.4	
Feasibility	3.2	2.8
Rank	9	26
In top 67% in terms of feasibility?	Y	Y
Evidence — min	1.6	
Evidence — 25th	2.3	
Evidence — median	2.6	
Evidence — 75th	2.9	
Evidence — max	3.4	
Evidence — mean	2.6	
Evidence — sd	0.4	
Evidence	2.8	2.6
Rank	21	27
In top 67% in terms of evidence?	Y	Y
Inequalities — min	2.0	
Inequalities — 25th	2.5	
Inequalities — median	2.8	
Inequalities — 75th	3.0	
Inequalities — max	3.8	
Inequalities — mean	2.8	
Inequalities — sd	0.4	
Inequalities	2.8	2.8
Rank	35	27
In top 67% in terms of inequalities?	Y	Y
Costs — min	2.0	
Costs — 25th	2.3	
Costs — median	2.5	
Costs — 75th	2.7	
Costs — max	3.1	
Costs — mean	2.5	
Costs — sd	0.3	
Costs	2.4	2.4
Rank	35	43
In top 67% in terms of costs?	Y	N
Outcomes — min	2.0	
Outcomes — 25th	2.5	
Outcomes — median	2.7	
Outcomes — 75th	2.9	
Outcomes — max	3.5	
Outcomes — mean	2.7	
Outcomes — sd	0.3	
Outcomes	2.7	2.9
Rank	39	13
In top 67% in terms of outcomes?	Y	Y
Confidence — min	2.5	
Confidence — 25th	3.0	
Confidence — median	3.1	
Confidence — 75th	3.2	
Confidence — max	3.5	
Confidence — mean	3.1	
Confidence — sd	0.2	
Confidence	2.8	3.1
Rank	59	35
In top 67% in terms of confidence?	N	Y
% missing scores across all members and all criteria	16%	0%

Reference distribution shown in the statistics columns (averaged over all members — min, 25th, median, 75th, max, mean, sd):

Dimension	min	25th	median	75th	max	mean	sd
Overall grade	1.9	2.5	2.8	3.0	3.6	2.8	0.4
Feasibility	1.7	2.5	2.7	3.1	3.6	2.7	0.4
Evidence	1.6	2.3	2.6	2.9	3.4	2.6	0.4
Inequalities	2.0	2.5	2.8	3.0	3.8	2.8	0.4
Costs	2.0	2.3	2.5	2.7	3.1	2.5	0.3
Outcomes	2.0	2.5	2.7	2.9	3.5	2.7	0.3
Confidence	2.5	3.0	3.1	3.2	3.5	3.1	0.2

Totals (label column): In top 20 levers in terms of overall grade? Total = 20 (hidden for summing 0); In top 67% for all five dimensions (a)-(e)? Total = 21 (hidden for summing 0); Satisfy both grade and dimension criteria? Total = 17 (hidden for summing 0).

Rank	Lever ID	IN or OUT	Lever	References	Overall grade	Overall grade Rank	In top 20 levers in terms of overall grade?	In top 67% for all five dimensions (a)-(e)?	Satisfy both grade and dimension criteria?	Feasibility	Feasibility Rank	In top 67% in terms of feasibility?	Evidence	Evidence Rank	In top 67% in terms of evidence?	Inequalities	Inequalities Rank	In top 67% in terms of inequalities?	Costs	Costs Rank	In top 67% in terms of costs?	Outcomes	Outcomes Rank	In top 67% in terms of outcomes?	Confidence	Confidence Rank	In top 67% in terms of confidence?	% missing scores across all members and all criteria
21b	En9	OUT	The Department of Housing and Urban Development would designate low income public housing as "smoke-free" to reduce childhood exposure to second hand smoke. Smoking would only be allowed in designated outdoor areas.		2.9	21	N	N	N	2.0	61	N	3.3	2	Y	3.0	16	Y	2.8	10	Y	3.1	7	Y	3.1	35	Y	4%
21c	H6	OUT	National health care quality organizations would develop and monitor standards of care for asthma-related hospitalizations. These asthma hospitalization standards would include: a) a joint physician and case-manager/social worker evaluation of the reason for admission, b) the family's completion of an asthma education program before discharge, c) providing the family with a simple written plan, in the family's language, regarding actions to be taken after discharge, including a follow-up appointment within one week of discharge, and d) phone follow-up by an asthma case-manager within three weeks of discharge.	F10 (15b, OUT) F12 (43f, OUT)	2.9	21	N	Y	N	2.8	26	Y	3.0	11	Y	2.8	27	Y	2.8	5	Y	2.8	20	Y	3.1	35	Y	0%

Distribution legend (averaged over all members):

Statistic	Overall grade	Feasibility	Evidence	Inequalities	Costs	Outcomes	Confidence
min	1.9	1.7	1.6	2.0	2.0	2.0	2.5
25th	2.5	2.5	2.3	2.5	2.3	2.5	3.0
median	2.8	2.7	2.6	2.8	2.5	2.7	3.1
75th	3.0	3.1	2.9	3.0	2.7	2.9	3.2
max	3.6	3.6	3.4	3.8	3.1	3.5	3.5
mean	2.8	2.7	2.6	2.8	2.5	2.7	3.1
sd	0.4	0.4	0.4	0.4	0.3	0.3	0.2

Summary column totals: In top 20 levers in terms of overall grade? Total = 20; In top 67% for all five dimensions (a)–(e)? Total = 21; Satisfy both grade and dimension criteria? Total = 17.

Rank	Lever ID	IN or OUT	Lever	References	Overall grade	Overall grade Rank	In top 20 levers in terms of overall grade?	hidden for summing	In top 67% for all five dimensions (a)-(e)?	hidden for summing	Satisfy both grade and dimension criteria?	hidden for summing	Feasibility	Feasibility Rank	In top 67% in terms of feasibility?	Evidence	Evidence Rank	In top 67% in terms of evidence?	Inequalities	Inequalities Rank	In top 67% in terms of inequalities?	Costs	Costs Rank	In top 67% in terms of costs?	Outcomes	Outcomes Rank	In top 67% in terms of outcomes?	Confidence	Confidence Rank	In top 67% in terms of confidence?	% missing scores across all members and all criteria
21d	H7	OUT	National health care quality organizations would develop and monitor standards of care for children who have had more than three asthma-related hospitalizations in a two year period. These standards would include case-management/social work services and primary care by a certified asthma provider. Care would include an examination by the certified asthma provider at least every three months and all necessary medications and equipment ordered by that provider.	F7 (30b, OUT)	2.9	21	N	0	Y	1	N	0	2.7	31	Y	2.9	16	Y	2.9	18	Y	2.8	5	Y	3.0	10	Y	3.2	21	Y	0%
21e	Ed4	OUT	National, state, and local school organizations would implement a broad-based asthma education program for teachers and children. This program would be part of the science curriculum in elementary school and high school. It would be a series of class lessons aimed at familiarizing students with the symptoms of asthma and with how to be helpful to a person with an asthma attack. The program would provide awareness of how common the condition is and how children with asthma can lead normal lives.	H10 (17b, IN) H11 (35a, OUT) F15 (54d, OUT)	2.9	21	N	0	N	0	N	0	3.2	12	Y	2.4	43	N	3.0	16	Y	2.7	17	Y	2.8	28	Y	2.8	57	N	9%

Distribution statistics (averaged over all members):

Statistic	Overall grade	Feasibility	Evidence	Inequalities	Costs	Outcomes	Confidence
min	1.9	1.7	1.6	2.0	2.0	2.0	2.5
25th	2.5	2.5	2.3	2.5	2.3	2.5	3.0
median	2.8	2.7	2.6	2.8	2.5	2.7	3.1
75th	3.0	3.1	2.9	3.0	2.7	2.9	3.2
max	3.6	3.6	3.4	3.8	3.1	3.5	3.5
mean	2.8	2.7	2.6	2.8	2.5	2.7	3.1
sd	0.4	0.4	0.4	0.4	0.3	0.3	0.2

Totals: In top 20 levers in terms of overall grade? = 20; In top 67% for all five dimensions (a)-(e)? = 21; Satisfy both grade and dimension criteria? = 17; hidden for summing = 0.

Rank	Lever ID	IN or OUT	Lever	References	Overall grade	Overall Rank	In top 20 levers?	In top 67% all five?	Satisfy both?	Feasibility	Feas. Rank	top 67%?	Evidence	Ev. Rank	top 67%?	Inequalities	Ineq. Rank	top 67%?	Costs	Cost Rank	top 67%?	Outcomes	Out. Rank	top 67%?	Confidence	Conf. Rank	top 67%?	% missing
26a	P6	OUT	Local health departments would conduct a case-by-case investigation of every asthma death. Feedback would be given to the patient's family and all health care parties involved. Information gathered in the investigation would be used to help prevent future deaths.	P7 (38, OUT)	2.9	26	N	N	N	3.1	14	Y	2.7	22	Y	2.7	37	Y	2.2	56	N	2.5	52	N	3.2	21	Y	1%
26b	F3	OUT	Specifically, the Federal government would provide subsidies for employer health benefits for working families earning up to 300 percent of the Federal poverty level. This subsidy would promote health insurance coverage for "working poor" families with access to employer-based health insurance.	F1 (2, OUT) F2 (7b, IN) F4 (33, OUT) F5 (5b, IN)	2.9	26	N	N	N	2.3	54	N	3.0	11	Y	3.2	10	Y	2.5	31	Y	3.1	8	Y	3.4	7	Y	1%
26c	O2	OUT	Specifically, the Federal government would provide funding for research on the feasibility and cost-effectiveness of asthma screening. This research would focus on: a) the development and evaluation of reliable and valid asthma screening tools b) the impact of screening on asthma treatment and outcomes and c) the feasibility of asthma screening in schools and as part of well-child health care visits.	O1 (1, IN) O3 (35c, OUT)	2.9	26	N	N	N	3.2	9	Y	2.8	20	Y	2.7	40	Y	2.3	46	N	2.7	35	Y	3.0	40	Y	8%

Rank	Lever ID	IN or OUT	Lever	References	Overall grade (mean)	Overall grade Rank	In top 20 levers in terms of overall grade?	In top 67% for all five dimensions (a)-(e)?	Satisfy both grade and dimension criteria?	Feasibility (mean)	Feasibility Rank	In top 67% in terms of feasibility?	Evidence (mean)	Evidence Rank	In top 67% in terms of evidence?	Inequalities (mean)	Inequalities Rank	In top 67% in terms of inequalities?	Costs (mean)	Costs Rank	In top 67% in terms of costs?	Outcomes (mean)	Outcomes Rank	In top 67% in terms of outcomes?	Confidence (mean)	Confidence Rank	In top 67% in terms of confidence?	% missing scores across all members and all criteria
29	F16	OUT	The American Boards of Pediatrics, Family Medicine, and other primary child health care providers would institute an asthma-specific core module in their national certification process for all their diplomates. These modules would include asthma diagnosis, evaluation of symptom control, indication for anti-inflammatory therapy, and key elements regarding patient education (e.g., medication and equipment use and avoidance of asthma triggers.) Diplomates who by examination score above a certain threshold would receive an asthma certificate that would qualify them as a certified asthma educator and experienced provider.	Ed8 (49b, OUT) F15 (54d, OUT) F17 (30c, OUT)	2.8	29	N	N	N	3.1	14	Y	2.2	52	N	2.2	57	N	2.4	43	N	2.7	32	Y	3.0	40	Y	1%
30a	En7	OUT	The American Academy of Pediatrics, working with other national groups, would form a taskforce to evaluate the tradeoffs of current national law limiting water temperature, i.e. – decreasing risks of burns versus reduction of exposure to mites among children with asthma and allergies.		2.8	30	N	N	N	3.5	2	Y	2.7	22	Y	2.6	44	N	2.4	37	Y	2.5	48	N	3.2	21	Y	5%

Column statistics legend (min, 25th, median, 75th, max, mean, sd):

Dimension	min	25th	median	75th	max	mean	sd	Total
Overall grade	1.9	2.5	2.8	3.0	3.6	2.8	0.4	
In top 20 levers in terms of overall grade?								20
In top 67% for all five dimensions (a)-(e)?								21
Satisfy both grade and dimension criteria?								17
Feasibility	1.7	2.5	2.7	3.1	3.6	2.7	0.4	
Evidence	1.6	2.3	2.6	2.9	3.4	2.6	0.4	
Inequalities	2.0	2.5	2.8	3.0	3.8	2.8	0.4	
Costs	2.0	2.3	2.5	2.7	3.1	2.5	0.3	
Outcomes	2.0	2.5	2.7	2.9	3.5	2.7	0.3	
Confidence	2.5	3.0	3.1	3.2	3.5	3.1	0.2	

Rank	Lever ID	IN or OUT	References	Lever
30b	F7	OUT		All private and public insurance programs would provide supplemental extended service benefits packages to cover all children with severe asthma (e.g. hospitalized, more than three ED visits per year) with limited co-payments. Extended services covered would include all tertiary care, an environmental assessment after repeated hospitalization, an annual evaluation by an interdisciplinary team to set treatment and management goals, and case-management services to coordinate care from multiple programs and sources in order to ensure that these goals are met.
30c	F17	OUT	F16 (29, OUT)	Accreditation bodies would require that all managed care organizations or integrated health care systems providing care for children with asthma have providers "experienced" in pediatric asthma in their networks. For instance, documentation of at least one annual visit with an "experienced provider" or in consultation with an "experienced provider" would be required for all children with asthma.

Metrics (distribution averaged over all members: min, 25th, median, 75th, max, mean, sd)

Criterion	min	25th	median	75th	max	mean	sd	Total	F7 (30b)	F17 (30c)
Overall grade averaged over all members	1.9	2.5	2.8	3.0	3.6	2.8	0.4		2.8	2.8
Overall grade (Rank)									30	30
In top 20 levers in terms of overall grade?								20	N	N
In top 67% for all five dimensions (a)-(e)?								21	N	N
Satisfy both grade and dimension criteria?								17	N	N
Feasibility averaged over all members	1.7	2.5	2.7	3.1	3.6	2.7	0.4		2.5	2.6
Feasibility (Rank)									46	38
In top 67% in terms of feasibility?									N	Y
Evidence averaged over all members	1.6	2.3	2.6	2.9	3.4	2.6	0.4		2.6	2.5
Evidence (Rank)									30	37
In top 67% in terms of evidence?									Y	Y
Inequalities averaged over all members	2.0	2.5	2.8	3.0	3.8	2.8	0.4		3.1	2.6
Inequalities (Rank)									13	46
In top 67% in terms of inequalities?									Y	N
Costs averaged over all members	2.0	2.3	2.5	2.7	3.1	2.5	0.3		2.5	2.4
Costs (Rank)									31	37
In top 67% in terms of costs?									Y	Y
Outcomes averaged over all members	2.0	2.5	2.7	2.9	3.5	2.7	0.3		2.8	2.7
Outcomes (Rank)									20	35
In top 67% in terms of outcomes?									Y	Y
Confidence averaged over all members	2.5	3.0	3.1	3.2	3.5	3.1	0.2		3.1	3.0
Confidence (Rank)									30	40
In top 67% in terms of confidence?									Y	Y
% missing scores across all members and all criteria									5%	10%

Rank	Lever ID	IN or OUT	Lever	References	Overall grade	Rank	In top 20 levers in terms of overall grade?	In top 67% for all five dimensions (a)-(e)?	Satisfy both grade and dimension criteria?	Feasibility	Rank	In top 67% in terms of feasibility?	Evidence	Rank	In top 67% in terms of evidence?	Inequalities	Rank	In top 67% in terms of inequalities?	Costs	Rank	In top 67% in terms of costs?	Outcomes	Rank	In top 67% in terms of outcomes?	Confidence	Rank	In top 67% in terms of confidence?	% missing scores across all members and all criteria
							Total = 20	Total = 21	Total = 17																			
33	F4	OUT	Specifically, Congress would amend Medicaid legislation to allow for presumptive eligibility of all children with severe asthma. Children diagnosed with severe asthma would be eligible for immediate coverage of medical care services under the Medicaid program, regardless of the status of their eligibility paperwork.	F1 (2, OUT) F2 (7b, IN) F3 (26b, OUT) F5 (5b, IN)	2.8	33	N	N	N	2.4	50	N	2.7	25	Y	3.1	13	Y	2.7	14	Y	2.9	15	Y	3.5	1	Y	10%
34	H8	OUT	National health care quality organizations, in collaboration with local asthma-surveillance units, would develop and monitor standards for the identification and evaluation of children who have survived asthma-related near death episodes. The evaluation and treatment plan for these children would include an environmental and social evaluation of the household, and monthly home visits by a health care provider for three months. These home visits would be designed to facilitate education, access to medications and equipment, compliance with medication regimens, and household environmental refurbishment.	F7 (30b, OUT)	2.7	34	N	N	N	2.5	43	N	2.5	37	Y	2.9	19	Y	2.7	14	Y	2.9	15	Y	3.2	16	Y	9%

Dimension distribution statistics (min / 25th / median / 75th / max / mean / sd):
- Overall grade: 1.9 / 2.5 / 2.8 / 3.0 / 3.6 / 2.8 / 0.4
- Feasibility: 1.7 / 2.5 / 2.7 / 3.1 / 3.6 / 2.7 / 0.4
- Evidence: 1.6 / 2.3 / 2.6 / 2.9 / 3.4 / 2.6 / 0.4
- Inequalities: 2.0 / 2.5 / 2.8 / 3.0 / 3.8 / 2.8 / 0.4
- Costs: 2.0 / 2.3 / 2.5 / 2.7 / 3.1 / 2.5 / 0.3
- Outcomes: 2.0 / 2.5 / 2.7 / 2.9 / 3.5 / 2.7 / 0.3
- Confidence: 2.5 / 3.0 / 3.1 / 3.2 / 3.5 / 3.1 / 0.2

Rank	Lever ID	IN or OUT	Lever	References	Overall grade averaged over all members (mean)	Overall grade Rank	In top 20 levers in terms of overall grade?	hidden for summing	In top 67% for all five dimensions (a)-(e)?	hidden for summing	Satisfy both grade and dimension criteria?	hidden for summing	Feasibility averaged over all members	Feasibility Rank	In top 67% in terms of feasibility?	Evidence averaged over all members	Evidence Rank	In top 67% in terms of evidence?	Inequalities averaged over all members	Inequalities Rank	In top 67% in terms of inequalities?	Costs averaged over all members	Costs Rank	In top 67% in terms of costs?	Outcomes averaged over all members	Outcomes Rank	In top 67% in terms of outcomes?	Confidence averaged over all members	Confidence Rank	In top 67% in terms of confidence?	% missing scores across all members and all criteria
					Total: 20				Total: 21		Total: 17																					
35a	H11	OUT	States would provide funding for all school nurses to be full time and to be trained as Certified Asthma Educators. These nurses would educate patients and other school staff and perform environmental monitoring. The nurses would be required to identify children with asthma, obtain peak flows, and develop care plans and/or appropriate referrals for those children.	Ed4 (21e, OUT) H10 (17b, IN) H12 (43c, OUT) F15 (54d, OUT)	2.7	35	N	0	Y	1	N	0	2.6	38	Y	2.5	37	Y	2.9	19	Y	2.5	26	Y	2.9	15	Y	3.2	16	Y	10%
35b	F6	OUT	All private and public insurance programs would provide supplemental preventive benefits packages, or coordinate existing benefits, to cover all children with asthma with nominal co-payments. Preventive services covered would include age-appropriate preventive medications, equipment necessary to deliver medications, three "asthma check-up" visits with a regular provider, an initial evaluation by an interdisciplinary team, and follow-up evaluations every 5 years thereafter.		2.7	35	N	0	Y	1	N	0	2.5	40	Y	2.5	37	Y	3.2	9	Y	2.4	37	Y	2.9	15	Y	3.2	15	Y	10%

Legend — statistics averaged over all members (min / 25th / median / 75th / max / mean / sd):

Dimension	min	25th	median	75th	max	mean	sd
Overall grade	1.9	2.5	2.8	3.0	3.6	2.8	0.4
Feasibility	1.7	2.5	2.7	3.1	3.6	2.7	0.4
Evidence	1.6	2.3	2.6	2.9	3.4	2.6	0.4
Inequalities	2.0	2.5	2.8	3.0	3.8	2.8	0.4
Costs	2.0	2.3	2.5	2.7	3.1	2.5	0.3
Outcomes	2.0	2.5	2.7	2.9	3.5	2.7	0.3
Confidence	2.5	3.0	3.1	3.2	3.5	3.1	0.2

Rank	Lever ID	IN or OUT	Lever	References	Overall grade	Overall Rank	In top 20 levers in terms of overall grade? (Total 20)	hidden for summing	In top 67% for all five dimensions (a)-(e)? (Total 21)	hidden for summing	Satisfy both grade and dimension criteria? (Total 17)	hidden for summing	Feasibility	Feasibility Rank	In top 67% in terms of feasibility?	Evidence	Evidence Rank	In top 67% in terms of evidence?	Inequalities	Inequalities Rank	In top 67% in terms of inequalities?	Costs	Costs Rank	In top 67% in terms of costs?	Outcomes	Outcomes Rank	In top 67% in terms of outcomes?	Confidence	Confidence Rank	In top 67% in terms of confidence?	% missing scores all members and all criteria
35c	O3	OUT	Specifically, public and private organizations would fund prospective research to evaluate the effect of intensive in-utero and early-life home environmental control (e.g. smoking cessation and elimination of mite and cockroach-infested areas) in preventing asthma in children at risk. Children at risk would include those who have a family history of asthma, were premature, or wheezed in the first year of life.	O1 (1, IN) O2 (26c, OUT)	2.7	35	N	0	N	0	N	0	3.1	13	Y	2.6	30	Y	2.3	51	N	2.5	26	Y	2.3	56	N	2.9	51	N	9%
38	P7	OUT	Local health departments would conduct a case-by-case investigation of every asthma near death. Feedback would be given to the patient's family and all health care parties involved. Information gathered in the investigation would be used to help prevent future emergencies for the patients in question.	P6 (26a, OUT)	2.6	38	N	0	N	0	N	0	2.5	46	N	2.6	27	Y	2.7	37	Y	2.7	12	Y	2.9	13	Y	3.0	40	Y	0%
39a	P2	OUT	In collaboration with state and local governments, the CDC would evaluate the availability and quality of asthma data from schools. This would include investigation of efforts to obtain asthma prevalence and morbidity estimates (e.g. school days lost) through school-based data collection.		2.6	39	N	0	N	0	N	0	2.8	30	Y	2.7	25	Y	2.5	47	N	2.1	59	N	2.6	43	N	3.2	16	Y	9%

Column header legend – "averaged over all members" distribution statistics (min / 25th / median / 75th / max / mean / sd):

Dimension	min	25th	median	75th	max	mean	sd
Overall grade	1.9	2.5	2.8	3.0	3.6	2.8	0.4
Feasibility	1.7	2.5	2.7	3.1	3.6	2.7	0.4
Evidence	1.6	2.3	2.6	2.9	3.4	2.6	0.4
Inequalities	2.0	2.5	2.8	3.0	3.8	2.8	0.4
Costs	2.0	2.3	2.5	2.7	3.1	2.5	0.3
Outcomes	2.0	2.5	2.7	2.9	3.5	2.7	0.3
Confidence	2.5	3.0	3.1	3.2	3.5	3.1	0.2

82

Rank	Lever ID	IN or OUT	Lever	References	Overall grade	Rank	In top 20 levers in terms of overall grade? (Total 20)	Satisfy both grade and dimension criteria? (Total 17)	In top 67% for all five dimensions (a)-(e)? (Total 21)	Feasibility	Rank	In top 67% in terms of feasibility?	Evidence	Rank	In top 67% in terms of evidence?	Inequalities	Rank	In top 67% in terms of inequalities?	Costs	Rank	In top 67% in terms of costs?	Outcomes	Rank	In top 67% in terms of outcomes?	Confidence	Rank	In top 67% in terms of confidence?	% missing scores across all members and all criteria
39b	En1	OUT	The Environmental Protection Agency and the Department of Housing and Urban Development would work with local asthma providers and advocacy groups to: a) establish minimum standards for "environmentally friendly" homes, b) provide funding for environmental remediation assistance to landlords and families, and c) educate landlords and building industry officials on the control of indoor environmental exposure for children with asthma.		2.6	39	N	N	N	2.5	46	N	2.7	22	Y	3.5	3	Y	2.3	47	N	2.5	47	N	3.0	40	Y	3%
39c	F9	OUT	Private and public payers of care would create incentive program(s) for providers who comply with preventive care standards. For example, health providers who comply with these standards would receive financial bonuses (e.g. cash and/or extra vacation days).		2.6	39	N	N	N	2.7	36	Y	2.4	43	N	2.1	58	N	2.5	26	Y	2.8	25	Y	2.9	55	N	10%

Distribution values (averaged over all members) for each dimension:

	min	25th	median	75th	max	mean	sd
Overall grade	1.9	2.5	2.8	3.0	3.6	2.8	0.4
Feasibility	1.7	2.5	2.7	3.1	3.6	2.7	0.4
Evidence	1.6	2.3	2.6	2.9	3.4	2.6	0.4
Inequalities	2.0	2.5	2.8	3.0	3.8	2.8	0.4
Costs	2.0	2.3	2.5	2.7	3.1	2.5	0.3
Outcomes	2.0	2.5	2.7	2.9	3.5	2.7	0.3
Confidence	2.5	3.0	3.1	3.2	3.5	3.1	0.2

Dimension	min	25th	median	75th	max	mean	sd	Rank	In top 67%?
Confidence (averaged over all members)	2.5	3.0	3.1	3.2	3.5	3.1	0.2	40	Y
Outcomes (averaged over all members)	2.0	2.5	2.7	2.9	3.5	2.7	0.3	46	N
Costs (averaged over all members)	2.0	2.3	2.5	2.7	3.1	2.5	0.3	51	N
Inequalities (averaged over all members)	2.0	2.5	2.8	3.0	3.8	2.8	0.4	43	N
Evidence (averaged over all members)	1.6	2.3	2.6	2.9	3.4	2.6	0.4	53	N
Feasibility (averaged over all members)	1.7	2.5	2.7	3.1	3.6	2.7	0.4	50	N
Overall grade (averaged over all members)	1.9	2.5	2.8	3.0	3.6	2.8	0.4	42	N

% missing scores across all members and all criteria: 18%

	value
Confidence	3.0
Outcomes	2.6
Costs	2.2
Inequalities	2.7
Evidence	2.1
Feasibility	2.4
Overall grade	2.6

hidden for summing: 0
Satisfy both grade and dimension criteria? Total 17, N
hidden for summing: 0
In top 67% for all five dimensions (a)-(e)? Total 21, N
hidden for summing: 0
In top 20 levers in terms of overall grade? Total 20, N

Rank	Lever ID	IN or OUT	References	Lever
42	F14	OUT		Congress and state legislators would enact legislation to penalize payers of care who selectively disenroll children who have high utilization of services, unless the disenrollment is for the purpose of transferring the patient to coverage under the SSI program. Some children with asthma are hospitalized and use the ED multiple times because of the baseline severity of their illness. Payers would be held accountable for financial and other costs to the child with asthma and his/her family as a result of the disenrollment.

Metric	En2 (Rank 43a)	En4 (Rank 43b)
IN or OUT	OUT	OUT
Lever	Public and private payers of care, with assistance from health departments, would fund an environmental assessment of the home of every child with asthma who meets certain criteria. The criteria would include several hospitalizations or a near-death episode. Inspectors certified by the Health Department would conduct the assessment. The results of this assessment, including the presence of smoking persons in the household, would be reported back to the health care provider and made part of the medical chart.	Congress and states would enact legislation to establish and fund environmental assessment and refurbishing programs for schools and day care centers. The assessment would concentrate on areas within schools where children with asthma are more likely to be affected (i.e., classrooms, indoor exercise rooms) and on schools in geographic areas where asthma outcomes are worse.
References	Other financing and regulation levers	Ed4 (21e, OUT) H10 (17b, IN) H11 (35a, OUT) H12 (43c, OUT)
Overall grade — min	1.9	
Overall grade — 25th	2.5	
Overall grade — median	2.8	
Overall grade — 75th	3.0	
Overall grade — max	3.6	
Overall grade — mean	2.8	
Overall grade — sd	0.4	
Overall grade	2.5	2.5
Overall grade — Rank	43	43
In top 20 levers in terms of overall grade?	N	N
In top 67% for all five dimensions (a)-(e)?	N	N
Satisfy both grade and dimension criteria?	N	N
Feasibility — min	1.7	
Feasibility — 25th	2.5	
Feasibility — median	2.7	
Feasibility — 75th	3.1	
Feasibility — max	3.6	
Feasibility — mean	2.7	
Feasibility — sd	0.4	
Feasibility	2.2	2.5
Feasibility — Rank	57	46
In top 67% in terms of feasibility?	N	N
Evidence — min	1.6	
Evidence — 25th	2.3	
Evidence — median	2.6	
Evidence — 75th	2.9	
Evidence — max	3.4	
Evidence — mean	2.6	
Evidence — sd	0.4	
Evidence	2.5	2.4
Evidence — Rank	34	45
In top 67% in terms of evidence?	Y	N
Inequalities — min	2.0	
Inequalities — 25th	2.5	
Inequalities — median	2.8	
Inequalities — 75th	3.0	
Inequalities — max	3.8	
Inequalities — mean	2.8	
Inequalities — sd	0.4	
Inequalities	2.9	2.9
Inequalities — Rank	19	19
In top 67% in terms of inequalities?	Y	Y
Costs — min	2.0	
Costs — 25th	2.3	
Costs — median	2.5	
Costs — 75th	2.7	
Costs — max	3.1	
Costs — mean	2.5	
Costs — sd	0.3	
Costs	2.4	2.3
Costs — Rank	43	47
In top 67% in terms of costs?	N	N
Outcomes — min	2.0	
Outcomes — 25th	2.5	
Outcomes — median	2.7	
Outcomes — 75th	2.9	
Outcomes — max	3.5	
Outcomes — mean	2.7	
Outcomes — sd	0.3	
Outcomes	2.6	2.6
Outcomes — Rank	41	41
In top 67% in terms of outcomes?	Y	Y
Confidence — min	2.5	
Confidence — 25th	3.0	
Confidence — median	3.1	
Confidence — 75th	3.2	
Confidence — max	3.5	
Confidence — mean	3.1	
Confidence — sd	0.2	
Confidence	3.1	3.2
Confidence — Rank	35	21
In top 67% in terms of confidence?	Y	Y
% missing scores across all members and all criteria	3%	5%

85

Rank	Lever ID	IN or OUT	Lever	References	Overall grade	Rank	In top 20 levers in terms of overall grade?	In top 67% for all five dimensions (a)-(e)?	Satisfy both grade and dimension criteria?	Feasibility	Rank	In top 67% in terms of feasibility?	Evidence	Rank	In top 67% in terms of evidence?	Inequalities	Rank	In top 67% in terms of inequalities?	Costs	Rank	In top 67% in terms of costs?	Outcomes	Rank	In top 67% in terms of outcomes?	Confidence	Rank	In top 67% in terms of confidence?	% missing scores across all members and all criteria
					2.5	43	N	N	N	2.4	50	N	2.3	49	N	3.1	11	Y	2.6	21	Y	2.8	31	Y	3.0	40	Y	21%
43c	H12	OUT	States would fund public health nurses trained in asthma education to cover all state certified childcare centers. These nurses would be required to identify children with asthma, obtain peak flows, and develop care plans and/or appropriate referrals for those children.	Ed4 (21e, OUT) H10 (17b, IN) H11 (35a, OUT) F15 (54d, OUT)																								
43d	Ed10	OUT	Professional associations in pediatrics and family practice, the NHLBI and other associations with an interest in asthma would mount an effort to raise asthma awareness among public policy makers. This asthma awareness campaign would target legislators and federal and state officials.	Ed9 (59, OUT)	2.5	43	N	N	N	3.3	6	Y	2.2	50	N	2.1	58	N	2.2	51	N	2.5	48	N	3.3	12	Y	13%

Distribution legend (averaged over all members):

Statistic	Overall grade	Feasibility	Evidence	Inequalities	Costs	Outcomes	Confidence
min	1.9	1.7	1.6	2.0	2.0	2.0	2.5
25th	2.5	2.5	2.3	2.5	2.3	2.5	3.0
median	2.8	2.7	2.6	2.8	2.5	2.7	3.1
75th	3.0	3.1	2.9	3.0	2.7	2.9	3.2
max	3.6	3.6	3.4	3.8	3.1	3.5	3.5
mean	2.8	2.7	2.6	2.8	2.5	2.7	3.1
sd	0.4	0.4	0.4	0.4	0.3	0.3	0.2

Totals: In top 20 levers in terms of overall grade? = 20; In top 67% for all five dimensions (a)-(e)? = 21; Satisfy both grade and dimension criteria? = 17

Rank	Lever ID	IN or OUT	Lever	References	Overall grade (mean)	Overall grade Rank	In top 20 levers in terms of overall grade?	In top 67% for all five dimensions (a)-(e)?	Satisfy both grade and dimension criteria?	Feasibility (mean)	Feasibility Rank	In top 67% in terms of feasibility?	Evidence (mean)	Evidence Rank	In top 67% in terms of evidence?	Inequalities (mean)	Inequalities Rank	In top 67% in terms of inequalities?	Costs (mean)	Costs Rank	In top 67% in terms of costs?	Outcomes (mean)	Outcomes Rank	In top 67% in terms of outcomes?	Confidence (mean)	Confidence Rank	In top 67% in terms of confidence?	% missing scores across all members and all criteria
43e	F11	OUT	The appropriate national and state agencies would provide accreditation for "Asthma Centers of Excellence" within local health care delivery systems according to more specialized standards. To obtain "asthma certification" hospitals would demonstrate adherence to special standards such as minimum number of providers with expertise in asthma (physicians, nurse practitioners, respiratory therapists, asthma educators, and case managers) and quality assurance protocols for asthma care.	H5 (49a, OUT)	2.5	43	N	N	N	2.9	23	Y	2.0	58	N	2.4	50	N	2.4	37	Y	2.7	35	Y	2.9	51	N	6%
43f	F12	OUT	Private and public payers of care would require accreditation to provide basic or more specialized asthma services as part of their condition for payment for these services. For example, all managed care organizations receiving payment for asthma hospitalization and ED care would be required to meet certain minimum patient education standards prior to the patient's discharge.	H6 (21c, OUT) H7 (21d, OUT) H8 (34, OUT) H9 (17a, OUT) F10 (15b, OUT)	2.5	43	N	N	N	2.1	60	N	2.1	55	N	2.6	44	N	2.5	26	Y	2.8	25	Y	3.2	21	Y	6%

Rank	Lever ID	IN or OUT	Lever	References	Overall grade averaged over all members							Overall grade	Rank	In top 20 levers in terms of overall grade?	hidden for summing	In top 67% for all five dimensions (a)-(e)?	hidden for summing	Satisfy both grade and dimension criteria?	hidden for summing	Feasibility averaged over all members							Feasibility	Rank	In top 67% in terms of feasibility?	Evidence averaged over all members							Evidence	Rank	In top 67% in terms of evidence?	Inequalities averaged over all members							Inequalities	Rank	In top 67% in terms of inequalities?	Costs averaged over all members							Costs	Rank	In top 67% in terms of costs?	Outcomes averaged over all members							Outcomes	Rank	In top 67% in terms of outcomes?	Confidence averaged over all members							Confidence	Rank	In top 67% in terms of confidence?	% missing scores across all members and all criteria
					min	25th	median	75th	max	mean	sd			Total		Total		Total		min	25th	median	75th	max	mean	sd				min	25th	median	75th	max	mean	sd				min	25th	median	75th	max	mean	sd				min	25th	median	75th	max	mean	sd				min	25th	median	75th	max	mean	sd				min	25th	median	75th	max	mean	sd				
49a	H5	OUT	Federal and state governments would fund the creation of certified "asthma-provider centers" within local health care delivery system(s). The asthma center staffs would include primary and specialist providers, asthma educators, and case managers. The centers would: a) be the hub for asthma education for providers within a geographic area, b) serve as specialty asthma referral centers for children with difficult-to-control asthma and children who lack an asthma-trained health care provider, and c)assist state and local asthma surveillance units in the collection of population-based asthma surveillance data for the communities they serve.	F11 (43e, OUT)	1.9	2.5	2.8	3.0	3.6	2.8	0.4	2.4	49	20	0	21	0	17	0	1.7	2.5	2.7	3.1	3.6	2.7	0.4	2.5	40	Y	1.6	2.3	2.6	2.9	3.4	2.6	0.4	2.1	55	N	2.0	2.5	2.8	3.0	3.8	2.8	0.4	2.8	27	Y	2.0	2.3	2.5	2.7	3.1	2.5	0.3	2.5	31	Y	2.0	2.5	2.7	2.9	3.5	2.7	0.3	2.7	32	Y	2.5	3.0	3.1	3.2	3.5	3.1	0.2	2.8	57	N	4%
														N		N		N											Y										N										Y										Y										Y										N	

Rank	Lever ID	IN or OUT	Lever	References	Overall grade averaged over all members							Overall grade	Rank	In top 20 levers in terms of overall grade? (Total = 20)	hidden for summing	In top 67% for all five dimensions (a)-(e)? (Total = 21)	hidden for summing	Satisfy both grade and dimension criteria? (Total = 17)	hidden for summing	Feasibility averaged over all members							Feasibility	Rank	In top 67% in terms of feasibility?	Evidence averaged over all members							Evidence	Rank	In top 67% in terms of evidence?	Inequalities averaged over all members							Inequalities	Rank	In top 67% in terms of inequalities?	Costs averaged over all members							Costs	Rank	In top 67% in terms of costs?	Outcomes averaged over all members							Outcomes	Rank	In top 67% in terms of outcomes?	Confidence averaged over all members							Confidence	Rank	In top 67% in terms of confidence?	% missing scores across all members and all criteria
					min	25th	median	75th	max	mean	sd									min	25th	median	75th	max	mean	sd				min	25th	median	75th	max	mean	sd				min	25th	median	75th	max	mean	sd				min	25th	median	75th	max	mean	sd				min	25th	median	75th	max	mean	sd				min	25th	median	75th	max	mean	sd			
					1.9	2.5	2.8	3.0	3.6	2.8	0.4									1.7	2.5	2.7	3.1	3.6	2.7	0.4				1.6	2.3	2.6	2.9	3.4	2.6	0.4				2.0	2.5	2.8	3.0	3.8	2.8	0.4				2.0	2.3	2.5	2.7	3.1	2.5	0.3				2.0	2.5	2.7	2.9	3.5	2.7	0.3				2.5	3.0	3.1	3.2	3.5	3.1	0.2			
49b	Ed8	OUT	Local asthma health care centers would hold CME-like courses for all primary providers who see pediatric patients with asthma. These providers would include family-physicians, pediatricians, nurse practitioners, respiratory therapists, and pharmacists. Based on the NHLBI National Guidelines, these programs would be simplified, adapted according to the same principles as patient educational programs, and certified by the Health Department.	H5 (49a, OUT)								2.4	49	N	0	N	0	N	0								3.5	3	Y								2.3	47	N								2.3	51	N								2.2	54	N								2.3	56	N								3.4	6	Y	10%
51	En6	OUT	State and local regulatory agencies would develop standards regarding higher water temperatures for commercial Laundromats. All Laundromats would be required to offer customers the choice of a higher water temperature. This would facilitate families' capacity to wash sheets and other materials for effective mite-control.									2.4	51	N	0	N	0	N	0								2.3	54	N								2.9	16	Y								2.8	32	Y								2.1	61	N								2.3	58	N								2.6	61	N	6%

Legend — distribution of values averaged over all members (min, 25th, median, 75th, max, mean, sd):

Dimension	min	25th	median	75th	max	mean	sd
Overall grade	1.9	2.5	2.8	3.0	3.6	2.8	0.4
Feasibility	1.7	2.5	2.7	3.1	3.6	2.7	0.4
Evidence	1.6	2.3	2.6	2.9	3.4	2.6	0.4
Inequalities	2.0	2.5	2.8	3.0	3.8	2.8	0.4
Costs	2.0	2.3	2.5	2.7	3.1	2.5	0.3
Outcomes	2.0	2.5	2.7	2.9	3.5	2.7	0.3
Confidence	2.5	3.0	3.1	3.2	3.5	3.1	0.2

Summary criteria totals: In top 20 levers in terms of overall grade? Total = 20; In top 67% for all five dimensions (a)-(e)? Total = 21; Satisfy both grade and dimension criteria? Total = 17. (hidden for summing = 0)

Rank	Lever ID	IN or OUT	Lever	References	Overall grade	Overall grade Rank	In top 20 levers in terms of overall grade?	In top 67% for all five dimensions (a)-(e)?	Satisfy both grade and dimension criteria?	Feasibility	Feasibility Rank	In top 67% feasibility?	Evidence	Evidence Rank	In top 67% evidence?	Inequalities	Inequalities Rank	In top 67% inequalities?	Costs	Costs Rank	In top 67% costs?	Outcomes	Outcomes Rank	In top 67% outcomes?	Confidence	Confidence Rank	In top 67% confidence?	% missing scores all members and all criteria
52a	Ed12	OUT	Health care providers would target parents of children with asthma for training as Certified Asthma Educators. These parents would then serve as local peer educators and role models.	F15 (54d, OUT)	2.4	52	N	N	N	2.7	31	Y	2.1	55	N	2.4	49	N	2.1	58	N	2.4	54	N	2.6	61	N	10%
52b	F8	OUT	Insurance programs would institute co-payment mechanisms that reward families who adhere to preventive care. For example, families would get reduced co-payments if they filled all preventive-medication prescriptions and attended all regular preventive visits.		2.4	52	N	N	N	2.2	57	N	2.3	48	N	2.0	62	N	2.5	26	Y	2.6	43	N	3.0	40	Y	4%
54a	P5	OUT	States would enact legislation requiring evaluation of all children for asthma as a prerequisite for school or day care enrollment. As part of the required school entry history and physical exam, parents would provide certification that their children have been evaluated by a licensed physician for the possible presence of asthma.		2.3	54	N	N	N	2.4	50	N	2.0	58	N	2.8	32	Y	2.4	37	Y	2.6	43	N	3.1	30	Y	12%

Stat legend for "averaged over all members" columns (Overall grade, Feasibility, Evidence, Inequalities, Costs, Outcomes, Confidence):

Column	min	25th	median	75th	max	mean	sd
Overall grade	1.9	2.5	2.8	3.0	3.6	2.8	0.4
Feasibility	1.7	2.5	2.7	3.1	3.6	2.7	0.4
Evidence	1.6	2.3	2.6	2.9	3.4	2.6	0.4
Inequalities	2.0	2.5	2.8	3.0	3.8	2.8	0.4
Costs	2.0	2.3	2.5 (median)	2.7	3.1	2.5	0.3
Outcomes	2.0	2.5	2.7	2.9	3.5	2.7	0.3
Confidence	2.5	3.0	3.1	3.2	3.5	3.1	0.2

Totals legend: In top 20 levers in terms of overall grade? (Total 20); In top 67% for all five dimensions (a)-(e)? (Total 21); Satisfy both grade and dimension criteria? (Total 17); In top 67% in terms of feasibility? (Rank 31).

Measure	H3	Ed11
Rank	54b	54c
Lever ID	H3	Ed11
IN or OUT	OUT	OUT
Lever	Health care delivery systems would institute electronic or other tracking mechanisms to identify patients with asthma who have not been evaluated for asthma in the past two years. Patients and providers would be notified that a follow-up evaluation may be necessary.	Standards for asthma education would include primary prevention education standards for pregnant women. Prenatal care providers would provide education to pregnant women regarding household risk factors for asthma (e.g. dust mites, smoke, pets, etc.) and the benefits of breastfeeding.
References	H2 (15a, IN) H4 (12, IN) F18 (61, OUT) F19 (58, OUT)	
Overall grade	2.3	2.3
Overall grade Rank	54	54
In top 20 levers in terms of overall grade?	N	N
hidden for summing	0	0
In top 67% for all five dimensions (a)-(e)?	N	N
hidden for summing	0	0
Satisfy both grade and dimension criteria?	N	N
hidden for summing	0	0
Feasibility	2.7	2.7
Feasibility Rank	31	31
In top 67% in terms of feasibility?	Y	Y
Evidence	2.0	2.5
Evidence Rank	58	34
In top 67% in terms of evidence?	N	Y
Inequalities	2.0	2.3
Inequalities Rank	62	51
In top 67% in terms of inequalities?	N	N
Costs	2.0	2.3
Costs Rank	62	47
In top 67% in terms of costs?	N	N
Outcomes	2.1	2.1
Outcomes Rank	62	60
In top 67% in terms of outcomes?	N	N
Confidence	3.2	3.1
Confidence Rank	21	30
In top 67% in terms of confidence?	Y	Y
% missing scores across all members and all criteria	3%	6%

Rank	Lever ID	IN or OUT	Lever	References
54d	F15	OUT	States would develop mechanisms for certification of asthma educators following national standards. For example, certification would be granted through examination or documentation of prior specialist training, or extended working experience with this population. Any health provider or allied health professional (e.g., health educators, social workers, case managers, respiratory therapists) may be eligible for this certification. A state board designated by the state health department would oversee the certification process and its implementation, including possible linkage of asthma education certification to reimbursement level of services.	Ed4 (21e, OUT) Ed12 (52a, OUT) H10 (17b, IN) H11 (35a, OUT) H12 (43c, OUT) H13 (60, OUT) F16 (29, OUT)

Overall grade averaged over all members

min	25th	median	75th	max	mean	sd	Overall grade	Rank
1.9	2.5	2.8	3.0	3.6	2.8	0.4	2.3	54

In top 20 levers in terms of overall grade? Total 20 — N
hidden for summing: 0
In top 67% for all five dimensions (a)-(e)? Total 21 — N
hidden for summing: 0
Satisfy both grade and dimension criteria? Total 17 — N
hidden for summing: 0

Feasibility averaged over all members

min	25th	median	75th	max	mean	sd	Feasibility	Rank
1.7	2.5	2.7	3.1	3.6	2.7	0.4	2.5	43

In top 67% in terms of feasibility? N

Evidence averaged over all members

min	25th	median	75th	max	mean	sd	Evidence	Rank
1.6	2.3	2.6	2.9	3.4	2.6	0.4	2.2	51

In top 67% in terms of evidence? N

Inequalities averaged over all members

min	25th	median	75th	max	mean	sd	Inequalities	Rank
2.0	2.5	2.8	3.0	3.8	2.8	0.4	2.3	51

In top 67% in terms of inequalities? N

Costs averaged over all members

min	25th	median	75th	max	mean	sd	Costs	Rank
2.0	2.3	2.5	2.7	3.1	2.5	0.3	2.4	37

In top 67% in terms of costs? Y

Outcomes averaged over all members

min	25th	median	75th	max	mean	sd	Outcomes	Rank
2.0	2.5	2.7	2.9	3.5	2.7	0.3	2.5	48

In top 67% in terms of outcomes? N

Confidence averaged over all members

min	25th	median	75th	max	mean	sd	Confidence	Rank
2.5	3.0	3.1	3.2	3.5	3.1	0.2	2.9	51

In top 67% in terms of confidence? N

% missing scores across all members and all criteria: 9%

Rank	Lever ID	IN or OUT	Lever	References	Overall grade	Rank	In top 20 levers in terms of overall grade?	In top 67% for all five dimensions (a)-(e)?	Satisfy both grade and dimension criteria?	Feasibility	Rank	In top 67% in terms of feasibility?	Evidence	Rank	In top 67% in terms of evidence?	Inequalities	Rank	In top 67% in terms of inequalities?	Costs	Rank	In top 67% in terms of costs?	Outcomes	Rank	In top 67% in terms of outcomes?	Confidence	Rank	In top 67% in terms of confidence?	% missing scores across all members and all criteria
58	F19	OUT	Accreditation bodies would require hospitals and managed care organizations to establish information systems to track and report on pediatric asthma patients or to have such systems ready within three years.	H2 (15a, IN) H3 (54b, OUT) H4 (12, IN) F10 (15b, OUT) F13 (63, OUT) F18 (61, OUT)	2.3	58	N	N	N	2.5	43	N	2.4	42	Y	2.2	56	N	2.2	54	N	2.3	55	N	3.2	16	Y	13%
59	Ed9	OUT	Professional pediatric and family practice associations would distribute the latest epidemiological and clinical trial data to their state and local affiliates as well as to state Medicaid associations, and HMOs. Such data would provide information on asthma prevalence and incidence, risk group profiles, and effective asthma-related therapies and interventions.	Ed10 (43d, OUT)	2.3	59	N	N	N	3.0	19	Y	2.5	37	Y	2.1	61	N	2.1	59	N	2.1	60	N	3.3	12	Y	12%
60	H13	OUT	Congress would create an "Asthma Peace Corps". This program would provide special training for nurses and physicians in asthma prevention and care and participants would serve as asthma educators and specialists to pay off their educational debt.	F15 (54d, OUT)	2.2	60	N	N	N	1.8	62	N	1.7	62	N	2.7	40	Y	2.2	51	N	2.5	48	N	2.5	63	N	9%

Column statistics (averaged over all members):

	min	25th	median	75th	max	mean	sd
Overall grade	1.9	2.5	2.8	3.0	3.6	2.8	0.4
Feasibility	1.7	2.5	2.7	3.1	3.6	2.7	0.4
Evidence	1.6	2.3	2.6	2.9	3.4	2.6	0.4
Inequalities	2.0	2.5	2.8	3.0	3.8	2.8	0.4
Costs	2.0	2.3	2.5	2.7	3.1	2.5	0.3
Outcomes	2.0	2.5	2.7	2.9	3.5	2.7	0.3
Confidence	2.5	3.0	3.1	3.2	3.5	3.1	0.2

Totals: In top 20 levers = 20; In top 67% for all five dimensions = 21; Satisfy both grade and dimension criteria = 17.

The "averaged over all members" header legend (min, 25th, median, 75th, max, mean, sd) for each dimension:

Dimension	min	25th	median	75th	max	mean	sd
Overall grade	1.9	2.5	2.8	3.0	3.6	2.8	0.4
Feasibility	1.7	2.5	2.7	3.1	3.6	2.7	0.4
Evidence	1.6	2.3	2.6	2.9	3.4	2.6	0.4
Inequalities	2.0	2.5	2.8	3.0	3.8	2.8	0.4
Costs	2.0	2.3	2.5	2.7	3.1	2.5	0.3
Outcomes	2.0	2.5	2.7	2.9	3.5	2.7	0.3
Confidence	2.5	3.0	3.1	3.2	3.5	3.1	0.2

Totals legend: In top 20 levers in terms of overall grade? Total = 20; In top 67% for all five dimensions (a)-(e)? Total = 21; Satisfy both grade and dimension criteria? Total = 17.

Rank	Lever ID	IN or OUT	Lever	References	Overall grade	Overall grade Rank	In top 20 levers in terms of overall grade?	hidden for summing	In top 67% for all five dimensions (a)-(e)?	hidden for summing	Satisfy both grade and dimension criteria?	hidden for summing	Feasibility	Feasibility Rank	In top 67% in terms of feasibility?	Evidence	Evidence Rank	In top 67% in terms of evidence?	Inequalities	Inequalities Rank	In top 67% in terms of inequalities?	Costs	Costs Rank	In top 67% in terms of costs?	Outcomes	Outcomes Rank	In top 67% in terms of outcomes?	Confidence	Confidence Rank	In top 67% in terms of confidence?	% missing scores across all members and all criteria
61	F18	OUT	Public and private purchasers of health care would evaluate claims for pediatric asthma cases to monitor quality of care. In areas where asthma is a reportable condition, health care payers and surveillance units would link their data systems to measure timing and adequacy of care. Results of these evaluations would be used to reward and/or sanction plans/providers.	P1 (21a, OUT) F9 (39c, OUT) F10 (15b, OUT) F12 (43f, OUT) F13 (63, OUT) F14 (42, OUT) F19 (58, OUT)	2.1	61	N	0	N	0	N	0	2.6	37	Y	2.1	53	N	2.3	55	N	2.3	50	N	2.1	59	N	3.1	29	Y	27%
62	En3	OUT	Local health and housing departments would establish regulations for reporting and fining of landlords who do not make medically necessary environmental improvement(s) to homes with children with asthma. Fines collected from landlords would be used to make the environmental improvements.	Other financing and regulation levers	2.1	62	N	0	N	0	N	0	1.7	63	N	1.6	63	N	2.7	40	Y	2.2	56	N	2.5	52	N	3.0	40	Y	4%

Rank	Lever ID	IN or OUT	Lever	References	Overall grade averaged over all members							Overall grade	Rank	In top 20 levers in terms of overall grade?	hidden for summing	In top 67% for all five dimensions (a)-(e)?	hidden for summing	Satisfy both grade and dimension criteria?	hidden for summing	Feasibility averaged over all members							Feasibility	Rank	In top 67% in terms of feasibility?	Evidence averaged over all members							Evidence	Rank	In top 67% in terms of evidence?	Inequalities averaged over all members							Inequalities	Rank	In top 67% in terms of inequalities?	Costs averaged over all members							Costs	Rank	In top 67% in terms of costs?	Outcomes averaged over all members							Outcomes	Rank	In top 67% in terms of outcomes?	Confidence averaged over all members							Confidence	Rank	In top 67% in terms of confidence?	% missing scores across all members and all criteria
					min	25th	median	75th	max	mean	sd			Total		Total		Total		min	25th	median	75th	max	mean	sd				min	25th	median	75th	max	mean	sd				min	25th	median	75th	max	mean	sd				min	25th	median	75th	max	mean	sd				min	25th	median	75th	max	mean	sd				min	25th	median	75th	max	mean	sd				
63	F13	OUT	Health departments would institute a grading scheme for health care systems and their "asthma-provider centers." The grading scheme would be based on national or state-level standards for asthma care and would promote compliance with those standards. The grading information would be provided to the public.	H5 (49a, OUT) H6 (21c, OUT) H7 (21d, OUT) H8 (34, OUT) H9 (17a, OUT)	1.9	2.5	2.8	3.0	3.6	2.8	0.4	1.9	63	20 N	0	21 N	0	17 N	0	1.7	2.5	2.7	3.1	3.6	2.7	0.4	2.1	59	N	1.6	2.3	2.6	2.9	3.4	2.6	0.4	1.8	61	N	2.0	2.5	2.8	3.0	3.8	2.8	0.4	2.1	58	N	2.0	2.3	2.5	2.7	3.1	2.5	0.3	2.0	62	N	2.0	2.5	2.7	2.9	3.5	2.7	0.3	2.0	63	N	2.5	3.0	3.1	3.2	3.5	3.1	0.2	3.1	30	Y	16%

Appendix G
Summary of Member Ratings for Committee Meeting

Population-Based Surveillance

General Strategy/Specific Lever	IN	OUT	
		≥ 4 Criteria	< 4 Criteria
Targeted Surveillance			
P4: State and local health departments would survey subgroups and/or geographic areas with worse outcomes.	X		
P6: Local health departments would investigate every asthma death.			X
P7: Local health departments would investigate every asthma "near" death.		X	
Broader Population-Based Surveillance			
P1: Congress and states would establish and fund local and state asthma-surveillance units.		X	
P5: States would recognize screening of all children entering school for asthma.			X
Development of Standards			
P3: CDC would require standards for asthma-related sentinel events and severity indicators.	X		
Research			
P2: CDC would evaluate availability and quality of asthma school-based prevalence and other data.			X

Environmental Assessment and Control

General Strategy/Specific Lever	IN	OUT
	≥ 4 Criteria	< 4 Criteria
Control/Assessment of Household Exposure		
En1: EPA and HUD work to establish home exposure standards, fund remediation, and educate builders and landlords.		X
En2: Health care payers would fund home assessment for at-risk children with asthma.		X
En3: Local health and housing departments would regulate and fine landlords who don't make medically necessary environmental improvements.		X
En8: Health care payers would extend DME coverage to items that reduce exacerbations of asthma.	X	
Control of School/Daycare Exposure		
En4: Congress and states would pass legislation to fund environmental assessment and refurbishment programs for schools and day care centers.		X
Control Exposure to Second-Hand Smoke		
En5: States would use tobacco taxes to fund free smoking cessation programs.	X	
En9: HUD would designate low-income housing as smoke-free.	X	
Control Water Temperature		
En6: State and local regulatory agencies would develop water temperature standards for commercial laundromats who in turn would be required to offer consumer choice.		X
En7: AAP would lead taskforce to evaluate pros and cons of national water temperature laws.		X

Health Care Organization and Delivery

General Strategy/Specific Lever	IN	OUT
	≥ 4 Criteria	< 4 Criteria
Disease-Management and Other Strategies to Streamline Asthma Care		
H1: Health care systems institute quality-improvement strategies in different health-care settings.	X	
H4: Tracking systems to identify "uncontrolled" patients based on pharmacy information.	X	
H2: Tracking system to identify "uncontrolled" patients based on health care use and school day lost information.	X	
H3: Tracking systems to identify patients with asthma who have not been evaluated in past two years.		X
Targeted Efforts for Patients with More Health Care Use or More Severe Asthma		
H9: National health care quality organizations implement education and follow-up standards for children discharged from the emergency department.	X	
H6: Implementation of standards for hospital-based and follow-up care for all hospitalized children.	X	
H7: Case management services and more frequent provider follow-up for all children hospitalized more than three times.	X	
H8: Case management and other extended services, including home visiting and environmental assessment and refurbishment, for children who experienced a "near death" event.	X	

Health Care Organization and Delivery (continued)

General Strategy/Specific Lever	IN	OUT	
		≥ 4 Criteria	< 4 Criteria
School and Community-Based Services			
H10: Establishing local combined health-care and school-based programs for asthma education, treatment and referral.	X		
H11: Training all school nurses as Certified Asthma Educators.		X	
H12: States fund asthma-trained public health nurses to cover certified child care centers.			X
Other Asthma-Specific Health Care Delivery Strategies			
H5: Federal- and state-funded "asthma provider" centers.		X	
H13: Congress establishes an "Asthma Peace Corps."			X

Education Levers

General Strategy/Specific Lever	IN	OUT
	≥ 4 Criteria	< 4 Criteria
Mass-Media Strategies		
Ed2: Government-sponsored national campaign with targeted efforts towards high-risk groups.	X	
Ed3: Athlete spokespersons campaign for improved awareness of asthma symptoms and treatment during sport participation.	X	
Family Strategies		
Ed7: Completion of asthma education course by all families of high-risk children.	X	
Ed6: Completion of asthma education course by all families with a newly-diagnosed child.	X	
Ed12: Train parents as "Certified Asthma Educators."		X
Development of Standards		
Ed1: National asthma and health care quality organizations set widely accepted standards for simple and minimum requirements for asthma education for different users.	X	
Ed11: Specific standards for primary prevention in pregnant women.		X

Education Levers (continued)

	IN	OUT
General Strategy/Specific Lever	≥ 4 Criteria	< 4 Criteria
Provider/Policymaker Education		
Ed8: CME-like asthma courses for all primary health care providers.		X
Ed10: Asthma awareness campaign targeting legislators and federal and state officials.		X
Ed9: Updates on asthma epidemiology and therapies for professional association affiliates, Medicaid associations, and managed care organizations.		X
Community-Based Efforts		
Ed5: Asthma volunteer organizations work with government agencies, health care organizations, and schools to implement certified asthma-education and smoking cessation programs.	X	
Ed4: School-based asthma education for all children and school staff.	X	

Financing and Regulation

General Strategy/Specific Lever	IN	OUT
	≥ 4 Criteria	< 4 Criteria
Universal Health Insurance		
F1: Private and public health care payers would provide affordable health insurance for all children.	X	
Incremental Expansion of Coverage		
F2: Increase Medicaid eligibility to include all children in families earning up to 300% of federal poverty level.	X	
F3: Federal government would provide subsidies for employer health benefits for families earning up to 300% of federal poverty level.	X	
F5: All private and public health care payers would provide uninterrupted insurance coverage to all children.	X	
Asthma-Specific Expansion of Coverage/Benefits		
F4: Congress would amend Medicaid to allow for presumptive eligibility of all children with severe asthma.		X
F6: All public and private insurance would provide supplemental preventive benefits package to children with asthma.	X	
F7: All public and private insurance would provide supplemental extended benefits package to children with severe asthma.	X	
Incentives for Preventive Care		
F8: Insurance programs would institute incentives that reward families adhering to preventive asthma care.		X
F9: Public and private payers of care would create incentives that reward providers who comply with preventive care standards.		X

Financing and Regulation (continued)

General Strategy/Specific Lever	IN	OUT
	≥ 4 Criteria	< 4 Criteria
Asthma Quality Standards through Accreditation/Payment		
F10: Accreditation of health care organizations would include evaluation of asthma care standards.	X	
F11: Accreditors would designate "Asthma Centers of Excellence" based on stricter standards.		X
F12: Public and private payers of care would require asthma accreditations as a condition of payment for asthma services.		X
F17: Accreditors would require providers of asthma care to have "experienced providers" in their networks.	X	
F18: Public and private payers of care would evaluate claims data to monitor quality of asthma care. Payers and surveillance units would link data systems to evaluate timing and adequacy of care.		X
F19: Accreditors would require health care organizations to establish computerized tracking systems.		X
Penalties for Disenrollment		
F14: Congress and states would pass legislation to penalize payers who selectively disenroll children with high service utilization.		X
Certification of Asthma Educators/Providers		
F15: States would certify asthma educators following national standards.		X
F16: Pediatric and primary care medical boards would institute asthma-specific core modules in their national certification process.		X

Other/Research

General Strategy/Specific Lever	IN	OUT	
		≥ 4 Criteria	< 4 Criteria
Broad Prevention Research			
O1: DHHS sponsored development and funding of research agenda for asthma prevention.	X		
Specific Prevention Research			
O2: Federal funding for research on feasibility and cost-effectiveness of asthma screening.		X	
O3: Public and private funding of research on effect of in-utero and early-life home environmental control on asthma outcomes.			X

Appendix H
List of 21 Revised Policy Levers for Final Vote During Committee Meeting

Original source lever(s) From List of 63	CATEGORY/ REVISED LEVERS	Tally of "yes" Votes	Final Policy Recommen-dation
	POPULATION-BASED SURVEILLANCE		
P1, 3, 4	Create national population-based asthma surveillance system. This includes establishing and refining standards, and funding state and local surveillance units.	8	10
P7	Make "asthma near death" a notifiable event at the federal level.	3	10
	ENVIRONMENTAL ASSESSMENT AND CONTROL		
En5	States would enact legislation to **use tobacco taxes and legal settlements to fund the creation and operation of a free,** Health Department-certified **smoking-cessation program.** Health care providers and school personnel would refer all smoking persons who live in a household with a child with asthma or who work in a school.	2	X[1]
En8	Public and private payers of care would **extend durable medical equipment coverage to items proven to reduce the exacerbations of asthma.** Such items would include mattresses, pillow covers and other items that play an important role in preventing exposure to known allergens. Funding for these items could also come from Title V (MCH). Influence insurance companies to cover these services through presentation of evidence. Focus on Medicaid as a more feasible program to expand DME coverage.	2	X
En9	Government agencies would **designate selected congregate housing as "smoke-free"** to reduce childhood exposure to second hand smoke. Smoking would only be allowed in designated areas.	1	X
New	Federal government would **extend incentives to states to create asthma "safe" communities,** through grants to aid in meeting the costs of environmental assessment and control interventions supported by evidence (e.g. including home assessments for high risk children, funding for pillows and mattress covers as DME, hot water options in Laundromats, congregate smoke-free housing), with grantee eligibility related to the adoption of certain safe community practices demonstration through compliance with pre-set environmental housing and other standards.	7	7

---

[1] An X indicates that this item received fewer than 3 votes and was therefore not included in the final 11 recommendations.

EDUCATION

Ed2, 3, 4	The US Department of Health and Human Services, in collaboration with other federal and state agencies and national asthma organizations, would promote early diagnosis, referral, and treatment of patients with asthma through an educational campaign in the national media. This campaign would familiarize the public with the symptoms of asthma and with how to be helpful to a person with an asthma attack. It would include a focus on sports participation and school-based asthma awareness, promoting an awareness of how common the condition is, and how children with asthma can lead normal lives. This campaign would also target high-risk populations, such as ethnic minorities and poor individuals with uncontrolled asthma.	6	9
Ed7	Health care providers would provide and track the **completion of an asthma education course by all families of high-risk children.** Health care payers would improve their reimbursement of education services and these services would be evidence-based.	6	2
Ed6	Health care providers would provide and track the **completion of a standardized basic-education course on asthma for any child newly diagnosed with asthma and his/her family.** The course would include information on symptoms, how to use medications and equipment, what to do in case of an attack, and avoidance of asthma triggers. Materials for the program would be simple, interactive, in the family's language, and at the appropriate reading-level. Health care payers would improve their reimbursement of education services and these services would be evidence-based.	1	X
Ed1	National asthma, provider, and quality assurance organizations would set simple, **minimal standards for the content of asthma education based on accepted evidence of efficacy.** Asthma education would be for patients/families, providers, and school personnel.	4	2
Ed5	Volunteer organizations with special interest and expertise in asthma (e.g., ALA, AAFA), with state and federal government support, would **promote implementation of Health Department-certified asthma education and smoking-cessation programs.** These organizations would work with health care organizations and schools in these implementation efforts.	1	X

IMPROVING HEALTH CARE DELIVERY ORGANIZATION AND DELIVERY

H10,11	DHHS in collaboration with other federal and state agencies and national asthma organizations would promote full-time school health services staff in every public school who will be trained to implement a coordinated school health program for school based asthma management which includes school health services, health education, healthy school environment, coordination with public and private health care systems and good options for physical activity.	8	8
H12	States would provide the funds for the provision of an **asthma-trained public health nurse to cover all state certified childcare centers.** These nurses would identify children with asthma, refer them to a knowledgeable provider, and develop care and implement asthma action plans for these children or directly work and train designated childcare center staff to perform these activities.	0	X
H1,2,4,6,7, 8,9	Health care providers would **implement disease management, care coordination, and other quality improvement strategies to 1) identify and track, and 2) improve care for their high-risk populations**	8	1,3

			in multiple settings. For example, through the implementation of education and follow-up protocols for all children discharged from the hospital or an emergency department for asthma, and/or more extensive case management and home visitation programs for children with 3 or more hospitalizations or a "near death" event.
OTHER/RESEARCH			
O1,2 Ed4,P2	5	11	The Department of Health and Human Services, in collaboration with other Federal and state health, environmental and housing agencies, would develop and implement a **broad national asthma prevention research agenda**. Research funding would be provided by the appropriate Federal agencies to investigate the feasibility, effectiveness, and cost-effectiveness of primary, secondary and tertiary community based asthma prevention programs, including behavioral health interventions. This would include support of demonstration efforts in areas such as: 1) providing asthma education to all children and staff in schools, 2) screening for asthma in school, 3) quality improvement and disease management strategies.
FINANCING AND REGULATION			
	5	4	Universal, guaranteed and continuous health coverage for all children is and should remain the national goal. Until then: 1)state Medicaid and SCHIP programs should make maximum use of existing options to extend coverage to uninsured children, including expanded coverage, continuous coverage and presumptive eligibility, 2) federal and state policies should create incentives for employees to offer affordable coverage to all workers with children, 3) federal and state policies should extend coverage to all children residing in the U.S., regardless of documentation status.
F1-5	7	5	Covered benefits for children with persistent asthma should be broad enough to permit all preventive and therapeutic interventions that have proven to be both effective and cost-effective, including spacers, pillows, mattress covers, etc.
F6,7	5	2	Provider compensation arrangements should be designed to reward the provision of outpatient preventive and management care, including teaching skills for patient self-management, and minimize the use of inpatient care.
F9	2	X	Accreditation bodies should require all ambulatory health care organizations to have systems in place for the monitoring of adherence to clinical guidelines for the management of pediatric asthma.
F10	3	6	Health care purchasers should require contracting ambulatory health care organization to meet evidence-based performance standards for the management of pediatric asthma.
F12	4	6,8,10	Public and private health care purchasers and other health care entities with whom they do business should ensure that the design of their health systems as well as the individual treatment and management decisions that are made recognize the coverage and payment obligations that will flow from heightened surveillance and the expansion of school based preventive services and management.
F13			

Appendix I
FEDERAL LEGISLATION RELEVANT
TO CHILDHOOD ASTHMA[1]

INTRODUCTION

Legislation related to childhood asthma was introduced and considered during the 106th Congress. This Appendix reviews that legislation. After summarizing the methodology used to carry out this review, we analyze those measures related to the authorization of new childhood asthma-related activities on which both House and Senate legislative action were completed as of the end of September 2000.

This analysis indicates that childhood asthma–related public policy constituted a significant focus of federal legislative activities during the 106th Congress. The result of this focus is significant new legislative authority on health care–related matters generally, and in the areas of asthma prevention, treatment, management, and research specifically. Furthermore, although community prevention activities beyond those specifically connected to the provision of health care did not receive as much attention, the legislation authorizes an important new study that could result in a greater national understanding of the role that community living conditions and the quality of public housing play in preventing and reducing asthma.

METHODS AND RESULTS

We used standard legislative research techniques to prepare this analysis, beginning with a computerized search of "Thomas" (the congressional website) on September 13, 22, and 28, 2000. The purpose of the search was to identify any legislation that specifically incorporated the terms "asthma", "childhood asthma", or "asthma" and "children." The search process was repeated several times, because it is customary for legislation that is pending to move rapidly and change status in the final weeks of the federal fiscal year.

This search process yielded 32 separate pieces of legislation introduced during the 106th Congress and containing the term "asthma." Because "Thomas" is designed to reflect congressional proceedings for which each phase of the congressional deliberation process results in a separately identifiable reported bill, in a number of cases several entries actually pertained to the same measure at different stages of the legislative process.

From the 32 asthma entries, we were able to identify the following principal measures introduced during the process:

1. Asthma Act (H.R. 1965)

2. Children's Asthma Relief Act (H.R. 2840, S. 805)

---

[1]This appendix appears as the appendix in Marielena Lara et al., *Improving Childhood Asthma Outcomes in the United States: A Blueprint for Policy Action*, Santa Monica, Calif.: RAND, MR-1330-RWJ, 2001. Dr. Sara Rosenbaum, one of the committee members, reviewed the legislation.

3. Asthma Awareness, Education and Treatment Act of 1999 (H.R. 1966)

4. Urban Asthma Reduction Act of 1999 (H.R. 875)

5. Children's Health Research and Prevention Amendments of 1999 (H.R. 3301)

6. Children's Public Health Act of 2000 (S. 2868)

7. Children's Health Act of 2000 (H.R. 4365)

8. Asthma Inhalers Regulatory Relief Act of 1999 (H.R. 136)

9. National Latex Allergy Awareness Week (H. Con. Res. 387)

10. National Alpha 1 Awareness Month (S. Res. 84)

11. Native Hawaiian Health Care Improvement Act Reauthorization of 1999 (S. 1929); reported in the Senate (S. 1929)

12. Pregnancy Discrimination Act Amendments of 2000 (H.R. 3861)

13. Public Health Osteoporosis Screening, Diagnosis and Treatment Act of 1999 (H.R. 2471)

14. Safe Medications for the Elderly Act of 2000 (H.R. 5140)

15. Clean Power Plant Act of 1999 (H.R. 2980)

16. Clean Power Plant and Modernization Act of 1999 (S. 1949)

17. Grants to Improve the Infrastructure of Elementary and Secondary Schools (H.R. 3071; H.R. 1820)

18. School Environment Protection Act of 1999 (H.R. 3275; S. 2109)

19. Public School Modernization and Overcrowding Relief Act of 1999 (S. 1454)

20. School Environment Protection Act of 1999 (S. 1716)

21. Comprehensive Health Access District Act (H.R. 298; H.R. 304)

22. Children's Health Insurance Accountability Act of 1999 (S. 636; H.R. 1661)

23. Social Security and Medicare Safe Deposit Box Act of 2000 (H.R. 4577)

24. Departments of Labor, Health and Human Services and Education and Related Agencies Appropriations Act, 2001 (H.R. 4577)

After briefly examining each of these introduced measures, we determined that they pertained to many of the issues that ultimately were included in final legislation. They also are an indication of the extent to which policymakers are broadly aware of the dimensions of the asthma problem and interested in identifying public policy interventions.

The areas addressed by the legislation covered the following matters: the general problem of insurance coverage for children; funds to ensure greater protections against asthma and access to basic asthma management and prevention in schools and communities; expansion of community health services related to asthma; and public education related to childhood asthma.

Substandard housing was one significant problem that did not appear to receive specific legislative recognition. The absence of asthma-related public housing legislation suggests either that the problem of substandard housing and its impact on asthma is not fully understood or that there is at present insufficient legislative support, even on an initial basis, for legislation aimed specifically at asthma-related housing improvements.[2]

A review of the legislation also suggests that the most active members of Congress on asthma-specific matters are from urban areas, where the asthma problem may be greatest and easiest to recognize. Almost all bills were introduced by members of Congress who represent urban districts, and several of the most important measures received bipartisan support from the start. This bipartisan approach to children's health issues has been a hallmark of Congress for decades.[3]

The legislative history for the bills is as follows:

- Various measures were referred to the Committees of Jurisdiction in both Houses.

- A series of separate measures pertaining to both childhood asthma and other matters was combined and reported in the form of omnibus legislation to authorize new activities related to childhood asthma. This legislation (The Children's Health Act of 2000, H.R. 4365) passed the House of Representatives on May 9, 2000.

- The House bill was then *engrossed in* (sent to and received by) the Senate, where several amendments were added on the Senate floor. Floor action occurred in the Senate on September 22, 2000.

- On September 27, 2000, the House of Representatives took up the Senate-passed version of the legislation and voted (395 to 25) to approve the bill as amended and send it to the President, who signed it into law on October 17, 2000.

A DESCRIPTION OF THE CHILDREN'S HEALTH ACT OF 2000

The Children's Health Act of 2000 is an omnibus piece of legislation that addresses numerous issues in child health. The asthma-related provisions of the Act consolidate a number of the smaller asthma-related measures introduced in the 106th Congress. The Act comprises 35 separate titles pertaining to children's health, as well as drug and mental-health services for youth.

Title V: Programs Related to Asthma

Title V of the Act (H.R. 4365, Title V), entitled "Asthma Services for Children," contains provisions of direct relevance to this analysis. It amends the Public Health Service Act (PHS Act) to create several new asthma-related program funding authorities.[4] In addition, Title V amends one existing PHS Act health program to strengthen its role in the prevention of asthma.

---

[2]This is not to suggest that there is not support for general improvements in public housing, only that the issue of housing reform tied specifically to asthma reduction did not appear in the legislation.

[3]Many of the most important measures to emerge around child-health improvement over the past 30 years have been strongly bipartisan. The most prominent examples of this bipartisanship in the area of children's health are the Medicaid reforms enacted between 1984 and 1990 and the creation of the State Children's Health Insurance Program (SCHIP).

[4]As of the end of September 2000, no final appropriations legislation for FY 2001 had been established. Therefore, it is not possible to report on the final funding levels for Title V.

Title V contains four subtitles: "Asthma Services," "Prevention Activities," "Coordination of Federal Activities," and "Compilation of Data."

Subtitle A: Asthma Services. The Act amends Title III of the Public Health Service Act to expand and strengthen preventive, treatment, and health and health-related asthma management services. Funds are authorized for five years, a typical length of time for health service programs authorized under the Public Health Service Act.

Title V of the Act adds a new Part P (§399L.) authorizing and requiring the Secretary to make awards to "eligible entities." An *eligible entity* is a "public or private non-profit private entity (including a state or political subdivision of a state) or a consortium of any such entities. (§399L(a)(3)). The awards are for the following purposes:

- To provide "quality medical care" for children who live in "areas that have a high prevalence of asthma" and who "lack access to medical care" (§399L(a)(1)(A)).

- To provide "on-site education" to parents, children, health care providers, and "medical teams" to recognize the signs and symptoms of asthma, and to train them in the use of medications to treat asthma and "prevent its exacerbations [sic]" (§399L(a)(1)(B)).

- To decrease "preventable trips to the emergency room" by making "medication" available to "individuals who have not previously had access to treatment or education in the management of asthma" (§399L(a)(1)(C)).

- To provide other services, such as smoking-cessation programs, home modification, and other direct and support services that "ameliorate conditions that exacerbate or induce asthma" (§399L(a)(1)(D)).

In making grants, the authorizing language (§399L(a)(2)) specifies that the Secretary may, but is not required to,[5] make grants that develop and expand certain projects:

- Projects to provide "comprehensive asthma services to children" in accordance with National Asthma Education and Prevention Program guidelines, including access to "care and treatment for asthma in a community-based setting" (§399L(a)(2)(A)).

- Projects to "fully equip" mobile health care clinics that provide "preventive asthma care," including diagnosis, physical examinations, pharmacological therapy, skin testing, peak-flow-meter testing, and other asthma-related health care services" (§399L(a)(2)(B)).

- Projects to conduct "validated asthma management education programs" for patients with asthma and their families, including "patient education regarding asthma management, family education on asthma management, and the distribution of materials, including displays and videos, to reinforce concepts presented by medical teams" (§399L(a)(2)(C)).

The Secretary may award grants under the law and must give preference to eligible entities that

> demonstrate that the activities to be carried out under this section shall be in localities within areas of known or suspected high prevalence of childhood asthma or high asthma-related mortality or high rate of

---

[5]Specific appropriations language may, of course, limit the Secretary's discretion with respect to the funding of these authorized activities.

hospitalization or emergency room visits for asthma (relative to the average asthma prevalence rates and associated mortality rates in the United States) (§399L(a)(2)(A)[sic]).

The Act specifies what can constitute "acceptable data sets" to include the following:

> Data from Federal, state or local vital statistics, claims data under title XIX [Medicaid] or XXI [State Children's Health Insurance Program (SCHIP)] of the Social Security Act, other public health statistics or surveys, claims data under title XIX or XXI of the Social Security Act, other public health statistics or surveys, or other data that the Secretary, in consultation with the Director of the Centers for Disease Control and Prevention deems appropriate (§399L(a)(2)(B) [sic]).

In their grant applications, eligible entities must identify how they will coordinate grant-supported activities with programs operated under Medicaid, SCHIP, the state Maternal and Child Health Services Block Grant, child welfare and foster care and adoption assistance programs, Head Start, WIC, local "public and private" elementary or secondary schools, or public housing agencies (§399L(b)).

Eligible entities that receive funding must provide evaluations of the operations and activities carried out under the grant. The evaluations must include a description of the health status outcomes of assisted children, an assessment of asthma-related health care utilization services, the collection, analysis, and reporting of data according to Centers for Disease Control and Prevention (CDC)-developed guidelines, and such other information as the Secretary may require (§399L(c)).

The level of authorized appropriations for the service program is "such sums as may be necessary" for fiscal years 2001–2005.[6]

Subtitle B: Prevention Activities. Subtitle B amends the Preventive Health and Health Services Block Grant (§1901 et seq. of the Public Health Service Act) to add a new category of authorized activities to establish, operate, and coordinate

> effective and cost-efficient systems to reduce the prevalence of illness due to asthma and asthma related illnesses, especially among children, by reducing the level of exposure to cockroach allergen or other known asthma triggers through the use of integrated pest management as applied to cockroaches or other known allergens (§1904(a)(1)(E), as added by Subtitle B, Title V).

Allowable expenditures under this new authority may include "the costs of building maintenance and the costs of programs to promote community participation in the carrying out of integrated pest management, as applied to cockroaches or other known allergens" (§1904(a)(1)(E), as added by Subtitle B, Title V).

No additional funding is authorized for this activity, since the Preventive Health Block Grant already is authorized on a "such sums" basis.[7]

Subtitle C: Coordination of Federal Asthma Activities. Subtitle C directs the Director of the National Heart, Lung and Blood Institute, through the National Asthma Education Prevention Program, to

---

[6]The determination of necessity under legislation such as this is made by Congress as part of the annual appropriations process. The legislation authorizes discretionary spending, rather than entitlement spending up to the level of need.

[7]Thus, the important question is whether FY 2001 appropriations levels for the Block Grant will be increased to reflect this new activity.

- Identify all federal programs that carry out asthma-related activities

- Develop, "in consultation with appropriate federal agencies and professional and voluntary health organizations, a federal plan for responding to asthma"

- Not later than 12 months after the date of enactment of the Children's Health Act, submit recommendations to the appropriate committees of Congress on ways to strengthen and improve the coordination of asthma-related activities of the federal government (§424B(a) of the Public Health Service Act, as added by Subtitle C, Title V).

The Director is required to include a representative from the United States Department of Housing and Urban Development in the NAEPP for the purpose of carrying out this federal study (§424B(a) of the Public Health Service Act, as added by Subtitle C, Title V). The legislation authorizes such sums as are necessary for carrying out the study.

Subtitle D: Compilation of Data. The Act amends the Public Health Service Act to require the Director of the CDC to conduct local surveillance activities to collect data on asthma prevalence and severity, and to compile and annually publish data on national childhood mortality related to asthma. The legislation authorizes such sums as may be necessary to carry out the activity.

CONCLUSION AND IMPLICATIONS

The Children's Health Act of 2000 contains important national public policy advances in childhood asthma prevention, treatment, management, and surveillance. The new grant-making authority under the law will provide funds to communities with a high prevalence of childhood asthma to improve the delivery and coordination of health. For communities with an elevated prevalence of asthma, it will provide funds for preventive education services. To the extent that state health agencies, consistent with the prevention provisions of the Act, redirect prevention health block grant funding and resources to pest-control activities, the legislation may yield increased investment in the control of known allergens. The identification of asthma as an area for the development of surveillance activities represents a statement of congressional concern regarding the importance of community health monitoring as part of an overall national policy strategy to reduce the impact and severity of asthma. Finally, the national policy study required under the Act will provide a framework for augmented activities that extend beyond the provision of health care and that reach critical issues related to the quality of housing and the community environment.

The Act is broad in scope and, if fully funded (that is, funded up to the level of defined need), could provide assistance to communities with high asthma prevalence. Inevitably, of course, actual funding may be below full need levels, as is the case with some PHS Act programs. Furthermore, the legislation does not contain improvements in insurance coverage for children, although legislation currently pending in Congress would, if enacted, increase the potential for coverage of particularly vulnerable groups of children, including recently arrived immigrant children. Nonetheless, the program represents movement toward a national asthma policy.

The success of the legislation will depend on more than funding levels. As drafted, the Act vests broad discretion in the Secretary of Health and Human Services to define key terms such as "high prevalence," "validated asthma management programs," "lack of access to management care," and other key terms that ultimately will determine who can qualify for funding and allowable uses of funds. In addition, the Secretary has discretion within the limits of the law (and such other limits that may be imposed as part of the appropriations process) to identify funding priorities, establish grant qualification standards, and determine what constitutes permissible expenditures and required inter-program coordination activities. How these decisions are made, the extent to which implementation includes consultation with experts in programs to which this new authority must relate, and the standards that emerge, will significantly further the ultimate reach of the program.

Finally, the legislation vests considerable discretion in states and communities to design interventions that meet local need. Evaluation of the program's components and states' responses to the legislation will be an important part of furthering the development of national asthma policy.

Appendix J
List of External Reviewers[1]

Agency for Healthcare Research and Quality
  Denise M. Dougherty, Ph.D.
    Senior Advisor, Child Health

American Academy of Allergy, Asthma & Immunology
  Gail G. Shapiro, M.D.
    President-Elect

American Academy of Family Physicians
  Herbert F. Young, M.D., M.A.
    Director, Scientific Activities Division
  Barbara P. Yawn, M.D., M.Sc.
    Director of Research, Olmsted Medical Center

American Academy of Pediatrics
  Robert A. Wood, M.D.
    Section on Allergy and Immunology Executive Committee
    Department of Pediatrics, School of Medicine
    The Johns Hopkins Hospital

American Academy of Physician Assistants
  Gabriel Ortiz, M.P.A.S., P.A.

American Association of Health Plans
  Peter Fitzgerald, M.Sc.
    Director, Quality Management and Health Services Research

American College of Allergy, Asthma & Immunology
  Emil J. Bardana, Jr., M.D.
    President
  William Storms, M.D.
    Asthma and Allergy Associates, Colorado Springs, CO

American College of Emergency Physicians

American Lung Association
  Fran DuMelle
    Executive Vice President

American Pharmaceutical Foundation
  William M. Ellis, R.Ph., M.S.
    Executive Director

---

[1]This appendix appears as part of Marielena Lara et al., *Improving Childhood Asthma Outcomes in the United States: A Blueprint for Policy Action*, Santa Monica, Calif.: RAND, MR-1330-RWJ, 2001.

American Public Health Association
  Larry K. Olsen, Dr.P.H., CHES
    Chair, School Health Education and Services Section

American Public Human Services Association
  Lee Partridge
    Director of the Health Policy Unit
  Erin Nagy
    Health Policy Analyst

American Thoracic Society
  William J. Martin, II, M.D.
    President

Asthma & Allergy Foundation of America
  Mary Worstell, M.P.H.
    Executive Director

Asthma and Allergy Network/Mothers of Asthmatics
  Nancy Sander
    President

Environmental Protection Agency
  Mary T. Smith
    Director, Indoor Environments Division

Health Care Financing Administration
  Timothy M. Westmoreland
    Director, Center for Medicaid and State Operations
  M. Beth Benedict, R.N., Dr.P.H., J.D.
    Social Science Research Analyst
    Office of Strategic Planning
  Beverly Koops, M.D.
    Medical Director, Health Care Financing
    Texas Department of Health

Health Resources and Services Administration
  Peter C. van Dyck, M.D., M.P.H.
    Associate Administrator
    Maternal and Child Health Bureau

National Committee for Quality Assurance
  L. Gregory Pawlson, M.D., M.P.H.
    Executive Vice President

National Heart, Lung, and Blood Institute
  Claude Lenfant, M.D.
    Director and Chair of the National Asthma
    Education and Prevention Committee
  Virginia Taggart, M.P.H.
    Division of Lung Diseases

Diana Schmidt
  Coordinator, National Asthma Education and Prevention Committee
Robinson Fulwood, Ph.D., M.S.P.H.
  Senior Manager, Office of Prevention, Education, and Control

National Institute of Allergy and Infectious Diseases
  Anthony S. Fauci, M.D.
    Director

National Institute of Child Health and Human Development
  Duane Alexander, M.D.
    Director

National Institute of Environmental Health Sciences
  Kenneth Olden, Ph.D.
    Director

Pacific Business Group on Health
  Cheryl Damberg, Ph.D.
    Director of Research and Quality

Society for Academic Emergency Medicine
  Brian J. Zink, M.D.
    President
  Jill Baren, M.D., FAAP
    Chair, Pediatric Interest Group
  Carlos Camargo, M.D., Dr.P.H.
    Assistant Professor of Medicine
    Harvard Medical School

University of California, Los Angeles; and RAND Health
  Arleen Leibowitz, Ph.D.
    Chair, Department of Policy Studies

U.S. Department of Education
  Debra Price-Ellingstad, Ed.D.
    Education Program Specialist
    Office of Special Education Programs

U.S. Department of Housing and Urban Development
  Warren Friedman, Ph.D., CIH

121

Appendix K
Voting Sheet for Suggestions from External Reviewers

Please return by e-mail or fax (310-451-6917) by 5pm EST Wednesday, January 17

ISSUE	OPTIONS	YOUR VOTE (choose only one)	COMMENTS
1. Environmental Assessment and Control in Schools (Recommendation 8)			
EPA and ALA noted this was missing from school recommendation. Both mentioned EPA's "Tools for Schools" program.	1. Leave as is (no mention of environmental control).		
	2. Explicitly state that the committee omitted this due to lack of evidence of importance of environmental triggers at school and/or of effectiveness of school environmental controls.		
	3. Include this as a sub-recommendation for recommendation 8 and refer specifically to EPA's "Tools for Schools" as the vehicle.		
2. Extension of Coverage to Non-citizen Children (Recommendation 4)			
One external reviewer and one committee member had doubts about political feasibility of including this in recommendation #4.	1. Leave as is (reference to non-citizens removed from main recommendation but left in sub-recommendation).		
	2. Remove from main and sub-recommendation but state under implementation options that coverage for non-citizens can be addressed at State level.		

3. Notifiable Events (Recommmedation 10.3)		
ALA does not support "notification systems" due to limited resources for other surveillance activities, and problems of confidentiality and appropriate medical follow-up.	1. Leave as is (see recommendation 10.3)	
	2. Delete recommendation 10.3 (notifiable sentinel events).	
	3. Limit rec 10.3 to death as only notifiable event.	
4. Limitation of asthma self-management education to kids with persistent asthma. (Recommendation 2)		
ATS says we should recommend self-management education for all children with asthma. APHA suggests that we further limit this to children at risk for acute asthma only.	1. Leave as is (persistent asthma only).	
	2. Add justification for why we limited this to kids with persistent asthma.	
	3. Extend recommendation to include kids at risk for acute asthma.	
	4. Extend recommendations to all children with asthma.	